NEW AGE
MEDICINE

A CHRISTIAN PERSPECTIVE ON HOLISTIC HEALTH

Paul C. Reisser, M.D.
Teri K. Reisser
John Weldon

GLOBAL PUBLIS

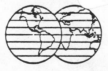

P.O. BOX 21788 • CHATTANOOGA, TN 37421

In Canada:
Purpose Products
P.O. Box 791
Aurora, Ont. L4G 4J9

Acknowledgment is made to the following for permission to reprint copyrighted material:

All quotations from Scripture, unless otherwise noted, are taken from the Holy Bible:
New International Version. Copyright© 1978 by the New York International Bible Society.
Used by permission of Zondervan Bible Publishers.

The excerpt on pp. 27-28 is from "Evolutionary Hymn" in Poems by C.S. Lewis, copyright ©1964 by the Executors of the Estate of C. S. Lewis. Reprinted by permission of Harcourt Brace Jovanovich, Inc.

The diagram on p. 57 is from Felix Mann, Acupuncture, illustrated by Frederic Metcalf, fig. 62, p. 153. Copyright © 1962, 1971 by Felix Mann. Used by permission of Random House, Inc.

Printed in the United States of America

Library of Congress Cataloging in Publication Data

Reisser, Paul C.
  New Age Medicine

  Includes bibliographies
  1. Holistic medicine-Religious aspects-Christianity.
I. Reisser, Teri K.   II. Weldon, John.   III. Title.

ISBN: 0-937931-26-8

Preface

The focus of our original book (*The Holistic Healers*, published in 1983), reflected in part the activities of the holistic health movement in the late 1970's. At that time, many of the movement's prominent speakers and writers proclaimed that holistic health would, within the next few years, make a dramatic impact upon the entire health care system of the Western world.

Needless to say, these expectations have gone unfulfilled. During the past decade, the practice of medicine has undergone significant changes –but not because of New Age thinking. The primary forces of change have been economic. The ever-increasing costs of manpower and new technologies have collided with the tightening purse strings of those who pay the bills. Seasoned physicians lament the "good old days" when their control over patient care was absolute. Now their decisions are molded by insurance company authorizations, government reviewers, patients who want to call more of the shots (or call off the shots), and the ever-present specter of malpractice suits if someone isn't happy with the outcome. Looming over this turbulent mix is the gathering storm of AIDS, which potentially could swamp the entire health care system within a decade.

In the midst of such turmoil, interest among physicians in the unorthodox therapies of holistic health has not been overwhelming, though not insignificant either. There has, however, been a marked increase in preventive medicine – in efforts to screen for cancer, discourage smoking, promote exercise, lower cholesterol and counsel against risky sexual behavior. These practical steps toward improved health have generally been overshadowed in the holistic health movement by an emphasis on unorthodox therapies and altering consciousness.

Holistic medicine has made some inroads among nurses (especially in the promotion of Therapeutic Touch), and a check of the yellow pages will invariably reveal a minority contingent of chiropractors who promote acupressure, applied kinesiology and other questionable pursuits. But for the most part, holistic medicine has remained squarely outside of the mainstream of professional standards of practice in the United States.

While holistic therapies have not taken American doctors and dentists by storm, they have continued to find plenty of new clients in the general public. In addition, the New Age movement –which is the primal force undergirding holism–has significantly increased its visibility. New Age themes weave through popular books, films and toys. Shirley MacLaine's books and TV miniseries "Out on a Limb" thrust reincarnation and spiritistic trance-channeling into the limelight. Discarnate spirits such as "Seth," "Lazaris," "Ramtha" and "Emmanuel" have become unlikely celebrities on TV and radio talk shows.

A three-year study by Stanford Research Institute International discovered that some twenty million Americans are "active in ideas ranging from astrology to yoga, to Transcendental Meditation, to parapsychology... to the study of the occult." Those engaged in such pursuits have been given a rather complimentary but misleading sociological designation: "experientially inner-directed."[1]

More recently, authors and speakers such as Dave Hunt, Johanna Michaelson and Constance Cumby have generated enormous interest among Christians in the New Age movement. The questions they and others have raised regarding the influence of New Age thinking upon the church have stirred up a storm of controversy. Yet although awareness of this movement has grown, discernment among Christians has remained marginal in the area of health care practices which are at one level or another hostile to biblical teaching (not to mention common sense).

More than half of the headquarters personnel of a highly-respected, worldwide evangelical organization have been treated with applied kinesiology, homeopathy and other holistic therapies. Guests on national Christian TV shows have endorsed similar practices. A bestselling Christian author uses and promotes a "Christian form" of acupressure, iridology, etc. The promoter of a healing program whose textbook was dictated by a "spirit guide" was given a friendly interview one Sunday morning at a well-known California church. We have continued to hear horror stories of churches embroiled in controversy, divided and quarreling after an alternative therapist wins some enthusiastic converts. A large midwestern Baptist church has been split down the middle over the practice of iridology.

Believers who would never dream of promoting the New Age movements are still capable of winning recruits to practices which express New Age thinking. Unfortunately, even when evidence indicates that a practice is incompatible with biblical teaching, not to mention scientific facts, the New Age therapy all too often gets the benefit of the doubt.

(An example: segments of *The Holistic Healer* were reprinted in three consecutive issues of the *Journal of Christian Nursing* in 1986. Our critique of Therapeutic Touch (included in this volume) elicited a significant amount of mail from Christian nurses who saw nothing wrong with this practice. The primary proponent of Therapeutic Touch, Dolores Krieger, claims that this technique manipulates a form of invisible energy, called prana—the existance of which is based squarely on Hindu mysticism. Obviously, there is nothing wrong with the compassionate touching of a patient. But there ought to be concern among Christian nurses over the notion that one's touch is unruffling or channeling prana, since doing so quietly validates the belief that "All is One" in the universe—and that we are all God.)

It is in response to these trends in our culture and the Christian community that *New Age Medicine* has been published. This book contains the entire text of *The Holistic Healers*, along with additonal material addressing the controversies raised by biofeedback, homeopathy and iridology. In addition, we have added some basic warnings to help guide those who are unsure whether a given therapy should be embraced or left alone.

Throughout much of the text from *The Holistic Healers* the term "New Consciousness" has been used in reference to what is now more commonly called New Age thinking. The two terms are essentially interchangeable.

It is our prayer that this book will help shed light on an area of ongoing confusion and turmoil among believers.

Paul C. Reisser, M.D.
Teri K. Reisser, M.S.
John F. Weldon, M.A., M.Div.
June, 1987

Other books written or coauthored by John Weldon:

Is There Life after Death? (Harvest House, 1977)
Close Encounters: A Better Explanation (Master Books, 1978)
Psychic Forces & Occult Shock (Global Publisher, 1986)
The 1980s Decade of Shock (Master Books, 1980)
Psychic Healing (Moody, 1982)
est (InterVarsity, 1982)
Playing with Fire (Moody, 1984)

Acknowledgements

For Paul and Teri Reisser this book has proven to be an impressively long project, and we appreciate the interest and encouragement of many friends who both cheered and harassed us to complete it.

The ongoing support of our parents –J.D. and Harriet Reisser, and Dick and Wanda Ketchum–has meant a great deal to us. We also wish to thank Chad and Carrie Reisser, who maintained good spirits when some bike rides and trips to the park were postponed while their parents worked toward the finish line.

John Weldon would like to acknowledge his indebtedness to the following people for their genuine kindness during the years this book was in preparation. Without their (and others') help, financial support and prayers, this and other projects would not have been accomplished: Jerry and Linda Beck, Ray Bentley, Bill and Loretta Bowers, Tal Brooke, Bob and Rita Cartwright, Steve and Susan Clark, Bill Counts, John Cully, Mike and Julie Dosh, Rosanna Gowan, Tim and Lynn Harris, Ron and Angel Jolivette, Hud and Nancy McWilliams, John MacArthur, Terry and Marlo Mulville, Paul and Elaine Newkirk, Don Schock, Peggy Smith, Mike and Karen Turk, John and Carol Whitehead.

Part I
The Holistic
Phenomenon

On a windswept Sunday morning in Los Angeles an articulate young Chinese woman surveys an audience of twenty-five hundred and asks for three volunteers. She has just concluded a message on the energy systems of the universe and their application to classical Chinese acupuncture. In return for braving the elements and leaving behind the Sunday *Times*, the audience now will be treated to a most unusual demonstration.

Two young women and an older man stand somewhat nervously onstage as the Chinese woman explains how applied kinesiology, or muscle testing, can demonstrate changes in one's life energy. With arms stretched forward and hands clasped, the first volunteer easily resists the speaker's efforts to pull her arms downward. Quickly, the speaker touches a few points around the head, and the startled volunteer's arms are pulled down without resistance. More points are touched, and strength returns as before.

The second woman is tested for arm strength. The speaker then places her hands in front of and behind the volunteer's head. Suddenly she passes her hands downward to the floor, like an illusionist making a magic pass over a box whose contents are about to disappear. After this is done, the second volunteer's arms drop with an apparently effortless pull. Then with a quick upward sweep of her hands, the Chinese woman restores the volunteer's strength as easily as she apparently drained it.

The third volunteer easily resists the arm pull, then waits as the woman walks behind him. Twice she gives a thumbs-up gesture behind him for the audience to see, followed by unchanged tests of strength. After a thumbs-down gesture, the surprised volunteer's arms drop with an easy pull. Another thumbs-up signal and complete resistance returns. The woman ends her presentation with an admonition to use such abilities for good. Later she informs a small group of bystanders that she did indeed lower the third volunteer's energy level simply by willing it to be done. "Is this magic?" one bystander asks.

"Only if you call it that," she answers.

The Chinese woman is Effie Poy Yew Chow, Ph.D., who has served as president of the East-West Academy of Healing Arts, as appointed member of the former National Advisory Council to the Secretary of Health, Education and Welfare, and as organizer of a major conference on holistic health and public policy in Washington, D.C.

Some time after Effie Chow's presentation, a man in a tailored three-piece suit slowly paces the same stage. He speaks in a detached yet pleading tone, as though his voice is about to be broken by the gravity of his subject. He tells the audience that the most important experience in life is the transformation of consciousness. One's normal, waking perceptions cannot understand and experience higher levels of consciousness which enable one to change time and matter, including the tissues of the body. The audience is implored to "tap the universal unpolarized consciousness," to "sense the totality of beingness," to "claim its inheritance."

After his message, a young woman asks the speaker to explain the significance of the blue rectangle that she and a friend saw floating back and forth over his head during his address. He does not know, but registers no surprise at the question. The speaker is W. Brugh Joy, M.D., product of the medical training programs of the University of Southern California, Johns Hopkins and the Mayo Clinic, former faculty member at USC School of Medicine and Good Samaritan Hospital, now director of the Sky High Ranch where consciousness transformation is on the daily agenda.

During the course of the day the audience will hear Norman Cousins, the former editor of the *Saturday Review*, deliver a defense of human potential and a warm account of his triumph over a deadly illness through laughter and the will to live. They will hear psychic healer Olga Worrall ask for science and religion to go steady and hopefully marry, and they will watch some unusual photographs, which show her fingertips glowing bright yellow with a blue flamelike corona as she "releases healing energy." Also on tap are the director of the UCLA Pain Control Unit, the chairman of the department of obstetrics and gynecology at Scripps Memorial Hospital in La Jolla, and the widow of Aldous Huxley.

Between speakers, members of the audience browse among exhibit booths, watching brain waves flicker in the EEG Mind Mirror, bouncing on a one-person exercise trampoline called the Sundancer, learning where to receive Laetrile, obtaining diagnostic portraits of the iris, checking blood pressure, hearing about acupuncture, biofeedback, hair analysis, stress reduction, vitamins and other assorted subjects. Some people meet informally in smaller rooms to participate in body movement therapies, experiment with biofeedback equipment, or meditate. A few dance to music pulsating through high-powered stereo equipment in the "health disco."

This audience of health professionals and lay people has assembled for the annual conference of the Center for Integral Medicine. This conference, like many others held in the United States every year, has a message: medicine is changing.

1
The Dawn of
Holistic Health

IN AN ECONOMIC FLIGHT of fancy one day a professor of molecular biophysics, Dr. Harold J. Morowitz, studied the catalog of a biological supply house and calculated the average value of a gram (roughly 1/30 of an ounce) of human being. Using the going rates for compounds such as hemoglobin ($2.95 per gram) and human DNA ($765 per gram), he arrived at the figure of $254.54 per gram of dry weight—that is, not including water. Using his own weight of 168 pounds and observing that humans are about 68 per cent water, he found to his delight that he was worth $6,000,015.44. The old formula which said that the raw materials contained in the human body—carbon, hydrogen, oxygen and so on—are worth about $.97 could finally be refuted. He was himself the Six Million Dollar Man!

Carrying this reasoning further, he concluded that even six million dollars' worth of purchases from the supply house was a miserable substitute for a human being. To assemble these into the substructures of cells (called organelles) would probably require at least six hundred billion dollars' worth of research and development, and to assemble the organelles into cells could not cost less than six thousand trillion dollars. Unfortunately, even a six-quadrillion-dollar cell culture would make a boring dinner companion. Dr. Morowitz was led to conclude:

How would we assemble the cells into tissues, tissues into organs, and organs into persons? The very task staggers the imagination. Our ability to ask the question in dollars and cents has immediately disappeared. We suddenly and sharply face the realization that each human being is priceless. We are led cent by dollar from a lowly pile of common materials to a grand philosophical conclusion—the infinite preciousness of every person.[1]

The psalmist arrived at the same conclusion as he pondered his being "woven" in his mother's womb: "I am fearfully and wonderfully made" (Ps 139:14 NIV).

For centuries scientists and poets alike have praised the human body as a marvel, a work of art, an engineering masterpiece, a mystery. Yet this same body, for all of its priceless intricacy, has a problem. Eventually, inevitably, something always goes wrong. It becomes colonized by microscopic invaders and maintains an uneasy truce, punctuated by battles called infections, not all of which are won. It is subject to cuts, bruises, burns and other insults by unyielding objects and forces. Its own cells may indulge in an orgy of uncontrolled multiplication and form a cancer, or turn against one another in the civil war called autoimmune disease. If it survives these or any of several other disasters, it still inevitably wears out and stops. There is no escape. The end point is universal, the world's only sure bet.

All human beings have stood on common ground in their experience of something going wrong with the physical body. Their inner responses to this—fear, hope, despair, resignation and, above all, the desire to feel better and be healed—have likewise varied little on the basis of race, creed or national origin. In what is felt to be the cause of the problem and what is done about it, however, there has been variety beyond description.

The Health Care System

For nearly all of human history the diagnosis and treatment of bodily malfunctions have belonged to the realm of the supernatural. Indeed, if a history of the world's medicine were to give equal time to each century of the past five thousand years, most of it would be a Who's Who of mystics, faith healers, gurus and shamans (the medicine man/priest of primitive societies). Only in the very recent past has the study of the human body been separated somewhat from a supernatural overlay. The process of observing, hypothesizing, experimenting and revising old ideas with new evidence—loosely what we call the scientific method—gained ground slowly (and often painfully) but eventually became pre-eminent in Western civilization as the primary approach to health and disease.

As a result, for most of us, responding to a physical problem (or attempting to prevent one) involves contact with a sophisticated complex of trained professionals and institutions which we call the health care system. This is the familiar world of doctors and hospitals, of x rays, drugs and surgery, the product of the scientific advances of the past few hundred years. The successes of this system are indisputable, and, at least until recently, its physicians and technologists enjoyed almost godlike status in society. Now, however, there are some cracks in Mount Olympus.

In the past several years the health care system (of the United States in particular) has come under a full-scale assault from an impressive number of critics in the media, government and the public at large. Most of these attack the *way* the system does (or does not) deliver the goods: it is seen as too expensive, unfair to the poor, sexist, racist, drug-pushing, time-consuming, and generally hazardous to one's health. While perusing the shelves of the public library one may encounter titles which would cause Marcus Welby to bury his stethoscope: *Don't Get Sick in America* by Daniel Schorr, *The Medical Offenders* by Howard and Martha Lewis, *Misdirected Medicine* by Dr. Sam McClatchie, *Medical Nemesis* by Ivan Illich, and *The Solid Gold Stethoscope* (subtitled "Warning: Your Doctor May Be Hazardous to Your Health") by Edgar Berman, M.D., to name a few.[2]

Western medicine is but one defendant in a more widespread popular prosecution of technology. The limiting of space exploration, the U.S. government's veto of the development of supersonic transports, and the daily battles over construction of nuclear power plants might all be considered examples of a revolt against the "destructive returns" of science. The once popular attitude that "if it can be done, it should be done" is being replaced by one giving social and ecological values a higher priority.

In medicine, the question of the limits of technology is for two reasons both thorny and poignant: first, because its subjects are human beings and not merely misbehaving cell cultures; and second, because so many physical (not to mention psychological) disorders remain complex mysteries, understood in only the crudest sense. We cannot approach a patient with the same detachment we might feel for a diseased tree or a mutant beetle. Humans come equipped with some very "nonscientific" feelings and needs, all of which are intensified if sickness prevails.

Furthermore, in spite of the general reluctance of the health care system to deal with it, the realm of the supernatural has never been far from the internist's examination table or the surgeon's operating theater. The need to feel relief is so powerful, the inability of scientific medicine to restore health so frequent, and the uncertainty generated by the one inevitable disease—death—so compelling, that the realm of faith, prayer and the paranormal is always close to the sickbed.

Here Western medicine is confronted with a new challenge. During the past few years a movement has been growing which argues that the health care system has lost touch with the human soul and spirit. This movement seeks to restore that broken relationship in the everyday practice of medicine. Its leaders call not just for an overhaul of the *way* medicine is practiced, but for nothing less than a radical revision of the underlying *thinking* about health and disease. This revision, it is said, necessarily includes reuniting modern medicine with its mystical traditions, as well as opening it to paranormal phenomena. The advocates of this transformation are fond of quoting Victor Hugo's observation that "nothing is as powerful as an idea whose time has come." They are convinced that the time has come for a "New Age" in medicine, for what they call *holistic health.*

The New Medicine
The holistic health movement at present defies simple definition. It is not represented by any single organization, group or type of practice, and it is continually being reshaped by its adherents. These include physicians and scientists with impressive credentials, chiropractors and osteopaths, psychologists and sociologists, healers and mystics, nurses and lay people, as well as an odd assortment of health "practitioners" whose ideas and techniques have varying degrees of credibility.

Organizations which promote or practice holistic health (by their own definition) range from storefront operations to associations with impressive budgets and conference schedules. San Diego's Association for Holistic Health and its metaphysical sibling the Mandala Society cohost an annual conference which draws over twenty-five hundred people with such speakers as Jonas Salk, Norman Cousins and Ruth Carter Stapleton. Some more modest groups possess little more than a post-office box number and a mailing list. The book *Wholistic Dimensions in Healing* by Leslie Kaslof lists eighty holistic organizations in the United States and Canada. These include conventional-sounding groups such as The Preventive Medicine Clinic (in Bellevue, Washington), as well as some bearing more interesting titles such as the Feathered Pipe Ranch (in Helena, Montana) or Naturo-Nutric Bionics (in Mound, New Mexico).[3]

It is impossible to estimate the total number of holistic practitioners and their patients at the present time, but we need not look far to see the movement's influence. Articles on the New Medicine or "universal energy" at times appear in such supermarket checkout staples as *Cosmopolitan* or *House and Garden.*[4] Courses on "yoga and health" are routine offerings at neighborhood recreational centers, and acupressure techniques are taught with increasing frequency as well. Lawmakers are obtaining their introduction to holistic health as they grapple with health-care legislation. The California Assembly's Health Committee, for example, has considered whether alternative health care is more cost effective than conventional medicine. A hotter issue, especially in California, is the legal status of some forms of alternative practice. Even the ill-tempered heroine of the comic strip *Broom Hilda* has been given some tongue-in-cheek advice by "The Holistic Doctor."

Despite the increasing visibility of holistic health, the movement is struggling to define itself, a task hindered both by its newness and its rapid growth. Sacramento Deputy District Attorney Dennis M. Warren, writing in the 1978 *Journal of Holistic Health* (published by San Diego's Association for Holistic Health), commented:

> In reality, the holistic approach is in its embryonic stage. There is no accepted consensus as to the scope of holistic practices, the role in medicine and society. There are no objective standards or guidelines for treatment. There is only a general philosophy of approach to health care. The rest is experimentation and individual implementation.[5]

Yet anyone who cares to read the literature of the movement and attend its meetings will begin to notice a distinct flavor, an over-riding viewpoint, a general philosophy (to use Warren's term) which is pre-eminent. The world view is none other than that of the "New Consciousness," a loose synthesis of various elements of mysticism, occultism, spiritism and animism, combined with concepts derived from modern paranormal research (i.e., parapsychology) and from the experiences of those who have experienced altered states of consciousness. Sometimes referred to as the human potential movement, the New Consciousness represents a sort of supernatural/psychic humanism which strives to bring about a radical transformation of thinking in society at large. The result, we are told, will be a New Age, referred to variously as the "Age of Enlightenment," the "Age of Aquarius," and other titles. Holistic health is, in essence, the banner under which the New Consciousness is making its move into the realm of health and medicine. Indeed, the holistic health movement does not appear nearly as concerned with changing the way medicine is practiced as it is with changing the fundamental orientation of people toward themselves, the universe, and especially the supernatural realm.

We should add at this point that the holistic movement is not the only setting in which health for the whole person is being promoted. Organizations which provide care or disseminate information without a New Consciousness slant (such as the network of Wholistic Health Centers founded in the Midwest by Dr. Granger Westberg) are becoming more vocal. Indeed, orthodox medicine is showing some interest in this direction, but its habits will not change overnight. Meanwhile, thousands of people are looking for alternatives to the care provided by organized medicine, and the New Consciousness at present is the most visible provider.

The time has indeed come for a refocusing of health care on the individual as a unique, whole, priceless being. The dimensions of mind and spirit have been isolated too much from the body, which is too often looked on as a biochemical machine. It is unfortunate, though, that for the time being the word *holistic* has been captured by those who are convinced that the New Consciousness holds the keys to health and wholeness.

We (the authors) wish to state at the outset a most important presupposition of our own. We view the Old and New Testaments as authoritative in all matters of life, including physical and spiritual health. Much of our critique of the current holistic health movement will therefore be derived from biblical principles. Our goal will be to identify the myriad forms of chaff which need to be separated from some very important wheat.

2
Ten Articles of Faith in the New Medicine

TO THE UNINITIATED, holistic medicine appears as a dizzying array of therapies which seem to have nothing in common. Indeed, the acupuncturist would share little with the aura reader, or the iridologist with the homeopathist, were there not a holistic health movement to unite such strange bedfellows. In order to comprehend the varieties of the New Medicine (as some call it), we must first understand some basic ideas which have been proclaimed repeatedly by the movement. We will summarize these presuppositions as ten widely accepted precepts. Some of these are truths which have been distorted or taken to extremes. Others present serious difficulties from a scientific or scriptural point of view.

The first two precepts are ones which we heartily endorse.

Precept 1
The whole is greater than the sum of its parts. One need spend little time at a holistic health conference before hearing of an over-

riding concern for the "whole person—body, mind, and spirit."
The word *holistic* (sometimes spelled *wholistic*) stems from the
Greek *holos*, meaning "whole" or "entire," a relative of the root for
our words *heal* and *health*. It was coined originally in 1926 by
South African Prime Minister Jan Smuts in his book *Holism and
Evolution*, a philosophical work not directly concerned with medicine. Indeed, Smuts's now-famous word has been applied to several fields (though usually in connection with the same cosmic
world view as in holistic health). One may, for example, hear references to holistic psychology, holistic law, holistic tennis and even
holistic sex.

Holistic health begins with the laudable premise that a human
being is more than a congregation of cells, a collection of tissues
and organs, or even a functioning (or ailing) physical body. A person is body, mind and spirit, a concept often illustrated by a drawing of three interlocking circles labeled with these terms and containing the word *unity* at the center.

While a few mechanists may quibble over the importance of
spirit in the above equation, only the most insensitive practitioner
could disagree with this basic idea. Even in a highly restricted sub-
specialty, where it is tempting to see the patient as an organ or two
which happen to have a human being attached, the perceptive
physician understands that the person who has the disease is as
important as the disease which has the person. No disorder occurs
in a vacuum.

This concept has two fundamental applications. First, the influence of attitudes, emotions and lifestyle on the origin and course of
disease is finally receiving some overdue attention. The consequences of self-destructive habits (such as smoking, overeating and
substance abuse) are obvious examples. The physical by-products
of long-term anger, anxiety and loneliness may include such diverse problems as headaches, peptic ulcer disease, irritable colon
syndrome, and possibly cancer.

Second, this precept lies at the heart of the Hippocratic Oath and
the more recent concept of a "patient bill of rights," both of which
call on health professionals to treat those in their care with dignity,

respect and compassion. This should strike a responsive chord in anyone who has felt like a serving of leftover turkey in a busy emergency room or an understaffed hospital. Humane and decent treatment of the sick should be a goal of responsible health-care providers (or anyone else), regardless of metaphysical orientation.

Precept 2

Health is more than the absence of disease. Vibrant health and terminal illness are extremes on a spectrum, and the holistic health movement emphasizes that no one should be content to be at a neutral, disease-free midpoint. Health means "feeling fine," being energetic, integrated, self-actualized and productive. George Leonard, once senior editor of *Look* magazine and author of *Education and Ecstasy*, argues:

> The conventional physician considers a person well if he has no symptoms and falls within the normal range in a series of diagnostic tests. Yet, this "well" person might smoke heavily, take no exercise, eat a bland, sweet, starch diet, and impress all who meet him as glum, anti-social, and emotionally repressed. To a New Medicine practitioner, such a person is quite sick, the carrier of what biologist René Dubos calls "submerged potential illness." In the New Medicine, the absence of overt disease is only the starting point, beyond which a whole world of *good health* beckons.[1]

Richard Svihus, M.D., who has served as president of the California Academy of Preventive Medicine, takes Leonard's statement a step further:

> Holistic Health is a state of being in which a person is integrated in all of his levels of being: body, mind, and spirit. . . . The attainment of this state of integration . . . brings into existence an entirely new person, different from what existed before, and at a new plateau of existence. I submit that this new state of being of an individual is a state of self realization or self actualization or enlightenment.[2]

Western medicine has been criticized for its preoccupation with disease and crisis intervention and for being content to return a patient from the negative end of the spectrum to a neutral, illness-free condition. In contrast to this, many holistic health proponents see themselves as promoting wellness, not merely combating illness. A wellness evaluation might include not only a review of previous illnesses or current symptoms, but also eating habits, recent (possibly stress-producing) life changes, personal goals, productivity and other dimensions of life.

This emphasis on wellness is certainly admirable and could be a more potent stimulus for disease-preventing behavior than fear of illness. Nevertheless, an important issue is that of who should be responsible for bringing about this condition. Western practitioners, especially those who grapple daily with the complexities of serious disease, may justifiably argue that their emphasis on the negative, on pathology, is entirely appropriate and that "wellness" is more the province of the psychologist, artist or theologian. Furthermore, in the holistic health movement, wellness has a tendency to be equated with enlightenment as understood in Eastern mysticism—involving altered states of consciousness in which psychic or supernatural experiences may occur.

Nevertheless, most physicians carry out routine checkups on patients for the purpose of detecting unsuspected disease, and large numbers of people seek medical advice regarding symptoms which prove to be heavily influenced by emotions and lifestyle. Doctors are thus logical candidates to give sound advice on habits which promote health. Ultimately, however (as we will discuss in more detail later), wellness is a matter of individual choice. This brings us to a third precept, which at its core is true but often is taken to extremes in the holistic health movement.

Precept 3

Individuals are ultimately responsible for their own health or disease. Holistic health proponents correctly insist that a patient participate actively in the healing process, rather than passively being a biological battleground. Some practitioners even dispense with the term *patient*, with its connotations of helplessness and control by outside forces. They prefer to use the term *client* and to think of the physician or healer as a coworker, teacher or guide.

This precept is interpreted in a variety of ways. The more conservative writers accurately criticize the "you heal me or I'll sue you" attitude of some patients, especially those who abuse their bodies for years and then present themselves to the nearest physician for a 50,000-mile overhaul. The more radical writers hold the patient ultimately responsible for *every* illness. Because of some misplaced attitude or lack of enlightenment, the person allows a disease to occur or even creates it. Svihus writes: "Now, disease is really a self-centered thing. Man is a creating entity and he manifests in matter his highest concepts of existence. Unfortunately, our highest concepts are not very high, because man tends to create cancer, heart disease, arthritis, wars, hatred."[3]

Often disease is seen as a learning experience specifically brought about by the body, or by the "universal intelligence," for the purpose of growth and evolution. Rick Ingrasci, M.D., writing in *New Age Magazine* (one of many New Consciousness periodicals) declares:

> In holistic health the emphasis is on the functional relationships among the various aspects of the whole person. Disease is understood to be a signal of disharmony or imbalance among the aspects of our being; it is looked upon as a teacher, a form of feedback which allows us to self-correct our life course and choose to grow in more positive, wholesome directions.[4]

Some people carry this idea to rather startling conclusions. Amy Wallace (coauthor of the best seller *The Book of Lists*) and Bill Henkin offer this eye-opening pronouncement in *The Psychic Healing Book*:

> The part of your body that becomes afflicted is communicating a message to you. For example, a disease of the sex organs bespeaks a reluctance to have sex; a sore throat or laryngitis points to a wish not to communicate; eye disease to a desire not to see what is going on around you or in your own life; shoulder and back pains suggest that you are carrying life's burdens on your shoulders or back.[5]

Most authors do not expose such naive thinking (it takes some fast talking to explain how herpes and gonorrhea come about because of a reluctance to have sex), but the concept of "illness as metaphor" is nevertheless popular in the holistic health movement. It contains some gaping holes in logic and offers little solace to those afflicted with serious illness. It is an especially poor explanation for cancer or other overwhelming disease in an infant or small child (not to mention disease in animals). Holistic metaphysics tends to fall apart in the neonatal intensive care unit or on the pediatrics ward.

The next precept, like the last one, has a core of truth to it. Unfortunately, it is often promoted with illogical fervor. When applied to the wrong disease, it can have disastrous consequences.

Precept 4

Natural forms of healing are preferable to drugs and surgery. Capitalizing on public disenchantment with the unsavory by-products of modern technology, as well as recent exposés of overprescribing and unnecessary surgery by some physicians, holistic health proponents proclaim the benefits of "natural" and self-healing. A recital of the latest adverse drug-reaction statistics is invariably included by at least one speaker at any holistic health conference. (The figures are nothing to sneeze at. One standard medical textbook indicates that five per cent of all hospital admissions are to some degree caused by complications of diagnostic tests or therapy).[6] More responsible spokespersons in the holistic health movement emphasize that conventional medicine has the decided edge in major trauma and emergency cases, but for other illness and prevention, they extol their favorite drugless, noninvasive therapies.

In this context holistic health is often tied with ecological awareness and with "universal life processes" which are inherently intelligent and self-correcting without intervention by technology. For example, John Thie, a California chiropractor and developer of Touch for Health (a popular blend of chiropractic and classical acupressure) writes:

The chiropractor believes that the innate intelligence that runs the body is connected to universal intelligence that runs the world, so each person is plugged into the universal intelligence through the nervous system. It is the job of the chiropractor to help this communication system, to insure that the body will function. He does this by working with the spine, the central core of the nervous system, the master system of the body. Then the body can take care of itself because there is no interference between the intelligences and the body.[7]

A positive by-product of the holistic health movement may be that of steering people away from a drug-oriented approach to life, but a less desirable result is the propagation of a peculiar logic which states that anything done without medications and surgery is by definition "natural." Healing methods which have no basis in reality or common sense, which openly defy well-established principles of biology and which in some cases tamper with dangerous realms of the occult, have acquired respectability by being referred to as natural. Similar semantic sloppiness occurs when the word *organic* is applied to certain (often overpriced) foods.

When a serious disease can be readily treated with medications or surgery, a patient's refusal to follow any approach other than a "natural" one might lead to a needless catastrophe. Most oncologists (cancer specialists) have had at least one case of a curable tumor which became hopelessly widespread while the patient pursued what seemed to be a more natural cure.

Precept 5

Any method of promoting health or preventing disease has the potential for being holistic, but some methods are more innately holistic than others. Many people in holistic circles have rightly observed that becoming healthy is a *process* which may involve a variety of therapies and lifestyle changes. Richard Svihus again: "The concept of Holistic Health doesn't imply the featuring of any particular treatment or diagnostic modality, and certainly doesn't imply a cover for a collection of questionable alternative practices. I don't think there is any one holistic therapy or any particular therapy which in itself is intrinsically holistic."[8]

Theoretically, the most highly trained subspecialist with the narrowest field of interest should be able to practice "holistically" if he or she keeps the patient's entire life in perspective. An example might be a cardiac (heart) surgeon conferring with patient and family together to determine preoperative concerns and postoperative support resources.

Nevertheless, in the holistic movement, there is an underlying (and sometimes overt) disdain for *allopathic medicine* (the generic term for conventional medicine), and a concurrent leaning toward therapies which are certainly alternative and usually questionable. Some of this learning represents an aggressive pragmatism: "Try *anything* if it might help." Beyond this, however, there exists a decided inclination toward practices which incorporate New Consciousness mysticism and occultism, both of which flourish within the holistic movement. The alternatives to Western medicine include the following.

a. Acupuncture, acupressure and their various derivatives (such as Touch for Health). Derived from ancient Chinese medicine and philosophy, these methods define disease as an imbalance in the flow of "energy." Treatment consists of stimulating the body at points which lie along lines of energy flow. (See part II.)

b. Biofeedback. A technique for bringing nonvoluntary bodily functions, such as heart rate, skin temperature and brain-wave patterns, under voluntary control, using instruments which measure and feed back information about these functions to the patient. Biofeedback has earned a positive reputation for treating migraine headaches and certain other physiological problems. However, some researchers, such as Elmer and Alyce Green of the Menninger Foundation, have also attempted to use biofeedback as a tool for inducing altered states of consciousness and psychic experiences.[9]

c. Chiropractic and osteopathy. Many practitioners of these familiar modes of therapy, which emphasize manipulation to correct spinal misalignments (or subluxations), are active in the holistic health movement. It is not unusual for chiropractors to use a variety of alternative therapies, such as acupressure, reflexology or

nutritional prescriptions, along with standard spinal manipulations. While a thorough study of chiropractic is beyond the scope
of this book, we will frequently make reference to situations in
which practitioners are delving into questionable or hazardous
territory.

   d. Homeopothy. A system founded by Samuel Hahnemann
(1755-1843), based on the concept that "like cures like." A substance which causes a symptom when given in large doses is said
to cure the same symptom when given in infinitesimal amounts.
The active ingredients in homeopathic remedies are so diluted that
they are said to work not according to laws of pharmacology, but
by infusing energy from their source to the patient. Ridiculed and
consigned to obscurity by nineteenth-century critics, homeopathy
is making a strong comeback, especially in England.

   e. Iridology. Limited exclusively to diagnosing illness, this system is based on the idea that a problem in any organ system becomes
visible as a localized change in color and texture of the iris (the
pigmented center of the eye). Recently popularized by Bernard
Jensen, a Los Angeles chiropractor and naturopath (a therapist
whose main tools are herbs and foods), Iridology has had proponents in Europe for decades. Diagnosis involves taking a detailed
color photograph of the patient's iris and comparing it to elaborate
charts which presumably are based on thousands of previous cases.
Iridology does not have overt metaphysical overtones (usually), but
Dr. Jensen has made his New Consciousness viewpoint clear in
articles and speeches.[10]

   It should be noted that iridology is never used as a diagnostic tool
by ophthalmologists. Furthermore, in one controlled study (conducted at the University of California and Veterans Administration
Medical Centers in San Diego, California), iridologists failed mis-
erably to diagnose end-stage kidney disease (their accuracy was less
than that of random guessing).[11]

   f. Massage and body-work therapies. These are a group of techniques which (with one exception) bear little relation to their
seamy counterparts on Hollywood Boulevard. All in some way
claim to release "energy imbalances," and most have overtly mys-

tical overtones. These therapies include:

Orgonomy (the exception noted above) was developed by Wilhelm Reich, who believed that illness arose when the free flow of "orgone" energy was inhibited in the body. This, conveniently, could be released by uninhibited sexual activity. (The word *orgone* was derived from *orgasm,* the improvement of which was a primary goal of Reichian therapy.) Reich also built and sold devices called orgone accumulators, which ultimately were frowned upon by the Food and Drug Administration and other authorities, leading to a jail term in 1957. Various Neo-Reichian therapies have been developed by his followers.

Functional integration, developed by physicist Moshe Feldenkrais, involves some one thousand physical and meditative exercises generally derived from yoga (indeed, it is sometimes called "western yoga").

Zone therapy bears certain similarities to acupressure, in that manipulation of certain zones of surface anatomy is said to have curative effects on distant organs. *Reflexology* is a form of zone therapy which concentrates on the palms of the hands and soles of the feet. It should be noted that these systems assume connections between distant parts of the body which bear no relation to known neurological pathways. An invisible flow is assumed here, as in many other holistic therapies.

Rolfing, also called structural integration, involves massage with a vengeance. In order to rearrange the body into a correct posture and relieve energy blockages produced by past traumatic experiences, trained Rolfers (a hundred fifty or so in the United States) subject their patients to deep pressures which are at times extraordinarily painful. Emotional release is said to occur, perhaps in the same way as when one hits one's head repeatedly with a hammer: it feels so good when stopped. Developed by the late Dr. Ida P. Rolf, it is based on some Reichian theories.

Do'in is similar in theory to acupuncture in that it strives for unhindered flow of "universal energy" through the body. It uses massage techniques rather than needles.

Shiatsu is similar to zone therapy, except that the areas manipulated are physically closer to the organ of interest.

Polarity therapy claims to balance the positive and negative polarities of the "life energy" flowing through the body by using relatively gentle massage, exercise and diet.

Bioenergetic analysis, a sort of psychotherapy through motion, deals with physical and emotional stresses through active and passive exercises. Some of these involve stretching the body in unfamiliar ways and observing both physical and emotional reactions to this stress.

g. Meditation, imagery and visualization. Meditation, invariably following one of the Hindu or yogic traditions, is almost universally extolled in holistic health as useful in relaxation, stress reduction, "normalization," and attainment of various states of enlightenment. Maharishi Mahesh Yogi's Transcendental Meditation, for example, has long advertised itself as a simple "non-religious technique" for bringing about desirable physical and psychological states. It has been actively promoted as an important tool in holistic health. Harold Bloomfield, M.D., a psychiatrist, TM initiator and author of the best-selling *TM-Discovering Inner Energy and Overcoming Stress*, has also published *The Holistic Way to Health and Happiness.* [12] He actively promotes TM at holistic conferences. TM is by no means the only meditation technique espoused in holistic health, but it is one of the most influential.

The use of visualization and guided imagery involves extending a meditative state to create a specific mental picture for diagnosis and healing. Irving Oyle, D.O., a colorful proponent of a "matter does not exist" worldview, teaches patients to visualize pleasant scenes in which a "guide" eventually appears. Supposedly generated by the patients subconscious, the guide may assume the form of a human or animal, providing insights into life's problems. There is cause for concern over what this guide represents, for the techniques bear a striking resemblance to the practice of contacting a "familiar spirit" as taught in standard occult texts. (More on this in chapter 8.)

Another approach is used by cancer therapists Stephanie and Carl Simonton of Fort Worth, Texas, who utilize a form of shamanistic imagery as an adjunct to standard therapies, training patient to envision their bodies fighting off malignant cells. Results in patients with widespread cancers were first reported as favorable, but have been questionable at best. [12a]

h. Nutritional therapies. The use of herbs, roots and foods of every description to cure and prevent illness has a long and colorful history which is beyond the scope of this book. It is not surprising that many advocates of various diets are jumping on the holistic bandwagon, given the movement's emphasis on drugless therapies and self-healing. Of somewhat more interest and concern is that New Consciousness metaphysics is finding its way into the corner health-food store, usually on the bookstand or the bulletin board. You might find a copy of *The Human Aura* nestled alongside Adele Davis, or announcements of acupressure workshops tacked next to listings of nutrition classes.

In addition, some writers in the health-food subculture are branching into more esoteric subjects. For example, Linda Clark, a nutrition reporter whose books are widely distributed in health-food stores, has also written *Help Yourself to Health*, [13] an innocuous sounding book (with daisies on the cover) which contains long passages of spiritism delivered with childlike enthusiasm. *Prevention Magazine* periodically features articles on alternative therapies such as acupressure or TM. For many, the search for a new diet may end with a new world view as well.

i. Psychic diagnosis and healing. This collection of practices, most of which are ancient, will later be considered at some length. When genuine they represent powerful, convincing and ominous demonstrations of contact with supernatural realms.

Psychic diagnosis includes any technique in which information about a patient is obtained without using ordinary methods of questioning, examination and reproducible data. *Psychometry*, for example, is the ability to gain information simply by holding an object (such as a key or coin) which belongs to an individual. *Clairvoyance* is "seeing at a distance," either while alert, meditating or in a trance. *Mediumistic* or *spiritistic diagnosis* is given by "spirit guides" who are said to be anxious to help ailing mortals. *Aura* readers claim to be able to see a multicolored radiation of energy surrounding a person. From its flickerings they diagnose physical and emotional problems.

Psychic therapies, as we shall see, are usually said to involve transfers (from healer to patient) of some form of "healing energy." This may take place through direct touch (laying on of hands), passing hands close to the body, or prayer in the most vague sense to an impersonal mass of cosmic energy. "Spirit guides" get into the act here, too, either by whispering the correct treatment into the ear of the healer or by taking direct charge of his or her body.

Psychic surgery, seen primarily in South America and the Philippines, is the hair-raising end point of occult medicine and the most difficult for Western, mechanistic thinkers to comprehend. Charges of fraud surround the Filipino surgeons, but too much has been observed at close range and on film in South America to dismiss this phenomenon as bloody magic tricks for primitive people. (See part III.)[14]

The next four precepts are spinoffs from the New Consciousness (or occultism), and either directly or by implication conflict with biblical teaching.

Precept 6

Health implies evolution. While *evolution* is one of the key words in the holistic glossary, it is not used in the usual Darwinian sense. It is instead a variation on some of Smuts's original ideas from the 1920s (his book was entitled *Holism and Evolution*). Drawing upon Smuts's book, the 1974 *Encyclopaedia Britannica* defines holism as "the philosophical theory based on the presupposition of emergent evolution, that entirely new things or wholes are produced by a creative force within the universe. They are consequently more than mere rearrangements of particles that already exist."[15]

Evolution in this context is both personal and global. Not only is the healthy, integrated individual said to be evolving toward "new plateaus of existence," but humanity as a whole is on the verge of a change which is more of a quantum leap than a gradual transition.

What we are all evolving toward, according to many holistic writers, is far more than just improved physical health or psychological well-being. We are, in fact, undergoing a psychic transformation, marked by an increasing awareness of the "creative force within the universe" and a blossoming acquaintance with its power. We are entering a New Age, which is to be marked by an awareness of realities beyond our everyday world, and medicine is but one of many fields which are on the verge of profound change. Arthur Freese, cowriter with Dr. Norman Shealy (a neurosurgeon and frequent speaker on the holistic health circuit), says in the introduction to a book entitled *Occult Medicine Can Save Your Life:*

> The now-people of our changing world have only recently begun to study the significance of this strange new era with its emphasis on the altered states of consciousness available to everyone, on a heightened sense of humane values, and on love and miracles and magic instead of technology and electronics and computers. Many of these new explorers like to emphasize these changes by giving this period its own name—the Age of Aquarius.[16]

The frequent, euphoric references to evolution by holistic speakers and writers are built upon a very weak (if not entirely imaginary) foundation. The basic tenets of biological macroevolution (that is, change from species to species) are now being publicly challenged on scientific as well as scriptural grounds. Even more tenuous is the idea that evolution necessarily implies improvement. C. S. Lewis playfully ridiculed this belief in his poem "Evolutionary Hymn," which begins:

Lead us, Evolution, lead us
   Up the future's endless stair:
Chop us, change us, prod us, weed us.
   For stagnation is despair:
Groping, guessing, yet progressing,
   Lead us nobody knows where.

Wrong or justice in the present,

Joy or sorrow, what are they
While there's always jam tomorrow,
While we tread the onward way?
Never knowing where we're going,
We can never go astray.[17]

Precept 7

To understand health and disease, we need an alternative model, one that is based primarily on energy rather than matter. The word energy is even more crucial in the holistic vocabulary than *evolution*, and it is invoked to explain practically everything from acupuncture to psychic surgery. We will devote an entire chapter to the concept of energy, for it represents an important effort to validate mysticism and occultism using scientific terminology.

In essence, many authors claim that Einstein's theory of relativity, which included the revolutionary idea that matter and energy were interconvertible (as graphically demonstrated by nuclear power), is directly applicable to biology. The idea that we are composed of "solid" matter is seen as an illusion, with profound implications. James Fadiman, who has served as director both of the Association for Transpersonal Psychology and the Institute of Noetic (that is, consciousness) Sciences, declares:

We are not primarily physical forms. We are primarily energy—or magnetic or whatever you like—forms around which matter adheres. Our primary nature is not physical. . . .

What happens is that as soon as you have that as a possibility, all kinds of data which have been battering themselves insensible against the old paradigm, fit. The laying-on-of-hands, obvious. Most paranormal data, obvious. . . . A lot of other nonphysical data becomes obvious as one does research and one finds better methods and so forth and so on.[18]

From this basic assumption—that we are energy appearing to be matter—flow a number of significant conclusions. Illness is not seen as a physical problem, but as an imbalance of energy in the body or as a by-product of unenlightened consciousness. Cure, likewise, belongs to the kingdom of the mind, which (given proper instructions) can manipulate the energies of its own body or of others.

Finally, we arrive at the classic conclusion of esoteric or occult thinking, that "all is one." It is said that we are not just independent blobs of energy, but an intimate part of the universal energy, the creative force of the universe, the universal consciousness, whose energy flows through us and unites us.

Psychologist Robert Gerard, appearing before a large audience at one of the first annual conventions of San Diego's Association for Holistic Health, led his listeners through a "mantra of unity" to help them experience the "unity of all things, the unity of our being." He then stated:

> I want you to start this way: look at each other and see the invisible. See that cosmic essence that runs within all of us, and know that this is the essence of the healing. For the essence of healing is in the capacity of both the healer and the healee [patient]. Be in touch with the quality of soul, with the quality of spirit. Be open to the energies of the universe, and allow these energies to flow through you.[19]

This concept of energy figures prominently in most Eastern religions and esoteric traditions. While not yet directly measurable, it is said to be demonstrable when one's consciousness is appropriately altered, using any of a variety of techniques. Most importantly, it is assumed that increasing scientific research into the paranormal or psychic realm (especially in the area of healing) will validate the existence and power of this energy and lead to a marriage of science and religion. Psychic healer Olga Worrall frequently expresses her hope that science and religion will one day "go steady, get engaged, and finally get married." Robert Gerard rhapsodizes on this possibility:

> The destiny of the human being is to become an integrationable [sic]: a mystical scientist, or a scientific mystic; a mystical healer, and a scientific healer; a mystical artist and a scientific artist —blending everything in ourselves, and recognizing that the energy that sustains the universe is one energy, which takes many different forms, but is still one energy.[20]

Precept 8

Death is the final stage of growth. The unbounded optimism of holistic health would rapidly wear thin in the face of human suffering, terminal illness and death, were it not for the recent emergence in some quarters of a more euphoric attitude toward the grave. Spearheaded by Raymond L. Moody, M.D., whose book *Life after Life* stimulated interest in the meaning of near-death experiences, a movement of sorts arose which viewed death not as an enemy, but as a passage into new realms of growth and understanding. The credibility of this movement was magnified by the involvement of Dr. Elisabeth Kübler-Ross, who has for years been recognized worldwide as an authority on the process of dying. (Her magnum opus, *On Death and Dying*, has long been recommended or required reading for health professionals.)

Since Kübler-Ross has had psychic experiences, including out-of-the-body travel and the acquisition of spirit guides, her thinking has changed significantly. Not many in her field of psychiatry, however, have followed suit. Needless to say, Drs. Moody and Kübler-Ross are favorites at the holistic health conferences.[21]

Precept 9

The thinking and practices of many ancient civilizations are a rich storehouse of knowledge for healthy living. In keeping with its general distaste for Western technology, the New Medicine tends to view certain ancient cultures as particularly holistic, integrated, in tune with the universal forces and rich in unique healing methods. For example, after decades of confinement to stuffy anthropology textbooks, the magic and rituals of shamanism have generated lively interest among investigators of paranormal healing. North and South American Indian healing practices, as demonstrated by medicine men such as Rolling Thunder, are being described as viable alternatives to the local physician.

Other cultures make similar contributions. Ancient China provides us with acupuncture, acupressure and its underlying Taoist philosophy. India's Vedantic Hinduism has made striking inroads into the West with yoga and meditation techniques and gives us its own concept of universal energy. Ancient Egypt is the source of numerous esoteric healing traditions, and its major sightseeing attraction has suddenly spawned a bizarre "technology" in pyramid power. Ancient Greece and Rome are of only marginal interest in the holistic health movement (despite the presence of Hippocrates), and ancient Judaism is virtually never mentioned, except in connection with its occult offshoot, the Cabala. Jesus is generally regarded as an enlightened healer whose miracles were powerful demonstrations of the energy available to us all.

In spite of the many healings recorded in the first century by the followers of Jesus, the teachings of the Old and New Testaments are not terribly popular in the New Medicine. The Bible proclaims such "unholistic" concepts as a personal God who intervenes in history, who is a Creator distinct from his creation, who holds human beings accountable to his standards of thought and behavior, and who judges humanity. Furthermore, the Scripture's announcement of Jesus' death as payment of the penalty for human rebellion, and of the need for individual repentance (not merely enlightenment) with disastrous consequences after death for not doing so, is blasphemy in the metaphysics of holistic health. The reason is obvious. The gospel of the New Consciousness may be reduced to two promises: (1) You will be gods (or God); and (2) You will not die.

It is interesting that these promises correspond with the temptations which were whispered to the first man and woman, as recorded in the opening chapters of Genesis. The bitter consequences of their seduction fill the remainder of the Old Testament and the subsequent history of the world. The fundamental incompatibility (*warfare* might be a better term) between the spiritual outlook which dominates holistic health and the teachings of Scripture is no small issue.

The last of the ten precepts reflects the concern of the promoters of holistic health for the legal and economic status of the New Medicine's assorted therapies.

Precept 10
Holistic health practices must be integrated into the mainstream

of life and health care through influencing public policy. The practitioners of alternative therapies are no longer content to work on the fringes of society and are now seeking widespread public acceptance. At stake here is not merely the issue of society's becoming more open-minded, but also such concrete questions as licensing, quality control, consumer protection, and payment for services by public and private medical insurance. California's lawmakers and its Board of Medical Quality Assurance have been studying a proposal to broaden the definition of *health practitioners* to include virtually anyone who adopts that title. This would, for all practical purposes, make practicing without a license a nonexistent issue. Some people are making a bid for reimbursement of various holistic therapies by programs such as Medicare, Medicaid and Blue Cross, which dispense millions of payments every year. Whether this occurs will have a great effect on the success of holistic health over the next several years.

3
Energy:
The Common
Denominator

IF HUMANITY SURVIVES long enough to produce a written history of the twentieth century, the focus of a final chapter will surely be the problem of energy. For a society now rudely awakened to the realities of finite resources, energy is fast becoming as precious as life itself. This was graphically demonstrated during the 1979 gasoline crisis when fights broke out among motorists awaiting their allotment of fuel. We use energy, we need it, and we will do nearly anything to obtain it. We can expect its importance in the near future to increase to almost godlike proportions.

Perhaps as a consequence, or perhaps as coincidence, we are seeing an exploding interest in another form of energy. This is not the product of familiar sources (the sun, the atom, the earth's deposits of crude oil), but rather what some believe to be an invisible, unmeasured, yet infinite energy which is the basis of all existence. In the New Consciousness and in much of holistic health, it appears under a variety of aliases, such as universal life energy, vital

forces, Ch'i, prana, bioplasma, para-electricity, and animal mag-
netism. We are told that, regardless of its name, this energy pervades everything in the universe, unites each individual to the cosmos, and is the doorway to untapped human potential. It is at the
root of all healing, all psychic abilities, all so-called miraculous
occurrences. It is what religions have called God. It is the crucial
link between science and religion, and it is awaiting our command.
In this chapter we will arbitrarily use the term *universal energy*. By
whatever name one chooses, however, it pervades the Mew Medicine, whether or not it pervades the universe.

Many heralds of holistic health somewhat naively link the idea
of universal energy to the latest developments in quantum physics.
They proclaim that the exploration of this energy will rank high on
the agenda for science in the future. Mary Coddington writes in her
book *In Search of the Healing Energy:*

> The findings of modern physics . . . have shattered the old mech-
> anistic, computerlike view of man's awareness. As a result, ex-
> ploring the true nature of man's consciousness has become a
> major occupation. It is, some feel, at the very cutting edge of cur-
> rent thought—thought that is giving birth to a new ontology or

Title	Origin
Prana	Hinduism
Ch'i (Ki, Qi)	Taoism and ancient Chinese medicine
Mana	Polynesian
Orenda	American Indian
Animal magnetism	Franz Anton Mesmer
The Innate	D. D. Palmer (founder of chiropractic)
Orgone energy	Wilhelm Reich
Vital energy	Samuel Hahnemann (founder of homeopathy)
Odic force	Baron Karl von Reichenback
Bioplasma	Contemporary Soviet parapsychologists
The Force	George Lucas (*Star Wars*)

science of being that recognizes man as a holistic unit of body-mind-spirit. . . . The healing energy, as we shall see, is an essential ingredient in this area.[1]

Actually, the idea of a pervasive life energy is very, very old. It has borne many names over the centuries, and to this day new labels are being applied to what is essentially the same concept. Some of these titles are listed on page 34, along with the person or system of thought associated with them.

Universal Energy: Some Basic Concepts

In the previous chapter we pulled some common threads out of the patchwork quilt of holistic health. In the same way we can extract a few basic ideas about universal energy out of the systems which promote it.

Universal energy is, first, said to be the basic fabric of everything, seen or unseen, in the universe. It is said to be omnipresent, flowing from the universe into living creatures, circulating within them in an orderly manner and ultimately flowing out again. It is not merely a *form* of energy, but it is *the* energy which is the basis for all life. Robert Giller, M.D., has stated:

This life force is manifested in our body—in our heartbeat, our respiration rate, our metabolism, our acid-base balance.

And to me, it's the same force that causes order in the universe; that causes the planets to circulate around the sun; that causes the change of seasons; that causes the tides; that causes, somewhere along the line, life itself.[2]

Here the New Medicine has appropriated for its own use the fundamental statement of the atomic age: $E = mc^2$. Einstein's famous equation, in simple terms, says that matter can be converted into energy and vice versa. The equation has been proved true, with spectacular results, under certain very special conditions. When matter is converted to energy under strict controls, we have nuclear power, a sizable (not to mention controversial) source of energy. An uncontrolled conversion of matter into energy, on the other hand, unleashes the fury of an atomic explosion.

Certain authors have seized upon this equation with misguided enthusiasm, making some "creative" applications to biology. Einstein, they insist, proved that matter and energy are the same thing. What we see as material objects (whether living or inanimate) are actually nothing more than congealed energy. Human beings are but one manifestation of universal energy. It does not merely flow through us; it is us. Traditional medicine, therefore, is portrayed as mechanistic, old-fashioned and pre-Einsteinian, because it treats the body as a material entity. The New Medicine, on the other hand, provides us with new ways to heal because it views the body as energy and manipulates energy to change the body.

One of the more vigorous proponents of matter-energy conversions in the human body is Irving Oyle, an osteopath and popular speaker on the holistic health circuit. In his book *Time, Space, and the Mind* he writes:

> The idea of the identity of energy and matter has enormous implications for all the healing professions. It gives us a theoretical basis from which to consider therapeutic methods such as acupuncture which purport to restore normal bodily states by manipulating the flow of cosmic energy. If energy and matter are indeed complementary states of a single entity, perhaps it is not unreasonable to hypothesize that by attention to the energy level, we can effect changes in the matter of the physical body.[3]

Oyle goes on to describe how, by manipulating consciousness through meditation and by contacting of inner guides, one can change energy and thus change matter, producing physical healing.

A major flaw in Oyle's thinking is duplicated among others who invoke Einstein as their inspiration. Oyle assumes that the conversion of matter into energy occurs in nature on a routine basis. He writes, for example, that a "simple way to observe the direct transformation of matter into energy is to watch a burning log disappear."[4] This statement would cause any high-school chemistry student (not to mention Einstein) to cringe. When a log burns, light and heat are produced and the mass of the log seems to disappear. Fortunately, however, a fireplace is not a nuclear reactor; the log is merely oxidized at a rapid rate, and one form of matter (wood) is converted to another (smoke and ashes). Energy is released as a by-product of the reaction, but not a single atom has been converted directly into energy. If it were indeed possible to transform a log into energy as defined by $E = mc^2$, the explosion would make a conventional atomic bomb look like a popgun.

The physical body is certainly changed by contact with energy (sticking one's finger into a candle will provide ample evidence), but to drag Einstein into the picture and claim that energy (universal or otherwise) in the human body *becomes* matter is completely erroneous.

The second assertion made about energy is that disease results from a blockage or imbalance in the natural flow of universal energy through the body. Most energy systems postulate some form of invisible circulation of energy which must be maintained to manifest health. The ancient Chinese, as we will show in the next three chapters, described an elaborate system of channels through which energy circulates. The Hindu concept of energy, known as prana, is said to flow through a series of psychic centers called chakras, which can be activated through meditation. D. D. Palmer, the founder of chiropractic, called universal energy the Innate and claimed that its flow through the nervous system could be blocked by spinal misalignments called subluxations. When a holistic practitioner makes reference to a blockage of energy as a cause of illness, he or she is invoking one or more of the systems we have mentioned.

Third, universal energy is said to be activated and channeled by a healer and may be used for both creative and destructive action. Nearly all therapies of the New Medicine presume to direct universal energy by one method or another, either by direct physical contact or by some form of invisible transfer from healer to patient. In ancient Chinese medicine, needles or other forms of stimulation at specific acupuncture points cause energy to flow more smoothly or to be rerouted. Classical chiropractic theory holds that spinal manipulations allow the Innate to flow more easily through the nervous system. Psychic healers, virtually without exception, claim to be channels for healing energy.

Rosalyn Bruyere, for example, a psychic healer and medium in Southern California (who served as technical adviser to Ellen Burstyn in the film *Resurrection*), claims to use a variety of energy systems in her work. As described by Ann Nietzke in *Human Behavior* magazine, "Bruyere uses her extensive technical knowledge of the chakra system, meridians, and pressure points to run healing energy into her patients by the laying on of hands. This is done by concentrating on the appropriate color and running that color into the appropriate location on the body."[5] Bruyere asserts that "the ability to heal is simply the ability to channel energy productively and cognize your thoughts and your intent without any vacillation."[6]

According to some authors, energy can be used destructively, as well as for healing. Descriptions of this process usually come from primitive societies, where "death magic" results in the "life force" being stolen from an enemy. Max Freedom Long, for example, in *The Secret Science behind Miracles* describes how kahunas (the priests/shamans of the early Hawaiian societies) induce spirit beings to rob an intended victim of mana, or life energy. Obviously such behavior is hardly holistic, and thus is condemned by modern energy manipulators. Nevertheless, such skeletons rattle in the closets of systems in which the line between science and magic wears thin.

A fourth proposition related to energy is that alterations in universal energy are the basis for all events which previously have been called supernatural or miraculous. If invisible energy can change or even become matter, we have a ready explanation for miracles. Healings, clairvoyance, psychokinesis and all other events of the paranormal realm merely represent the activity of universal energy, usually under the influence of an enlightened or psychic individual. Dr. William Tiller, professor of materials science at Stanford University and a theoretician in the holistic health movement, sets forth some of the implications of universal energy:

> One is that there are new energies which we have never dealt with before in physics; second, that we have within our organisms sensory capacities for cognition of these energies; third, at some level of the universe, we are all connected . . . ; fourth,

time, space, and matter are all mutable. We can perceive events out of our fixed location in space: that's remote viewing. We can perceive events out of our fixed location in time: that's precognition. Some people can materialize and dematerialize objects. If one can do it, eventually all will do it.[7]

Once we begin to understand and use the energy which is available to all of us, the miraculous will become commonplace, and the religion of the past will become the science of the future. Thus say the prophets of the New Age.

This brings us to our last, but not least, idea about energy. Universal energy is what religions have called God. Since man and woman consist of universal energy which has assumed material form, they are God. This is the bottom line, the fundamental message of many holistic healers, and one of the key doctrines of the New Consciousness. The concept of universal energy is the crucial link in the chain between science and religion which many are so anxious to forge. If this energy is both the stuff of which we are all made and the life force which flows through us every day, if it manifests intelligence and love, and if it guides our physical and psychic evolution, then it can be nothing less than God.

Holistic healers are more than willing to proclaim this idea. Rosalyn Bruyere, for example, states quite plainly that "for me, the terms God and energy are interchangeable. God is all there is, and energy is all there is, and I can't separate the two."[8]

Evarts Loomis, M.D., addressing one of the first conferences of San Diego's Association for Holistic Health in 1976, asserted that "expanded consciousness depends upon the inflow of primal energies variously referred to by different cultures as THE LOGOS, PRANA, CHI, BUDDHA NATURE, NATURE, THE WORD, THE HOLY SPIRIT, COSMIC ENERGY, etc. Who can say that these words are not synonymous?"[9]

The same conference received an invocation from the Reverend Jack Lindquist, then president of the San Diego Ecumenical Council, who read from the Gospel of Mark the story of Jesus' healing of a paralytic man. Lindquist expressed hope in his prayer that the "healing power of the universe, which many people call God," would move through the conference.

Some of these same people fervently declare that man is divine, that each of us is God, since man, God and energy are said to be one and the same. Psychologist Jack Gibb said it plainly: "The absolute assumption that a lot of us are making in the holistic health movement is that all of the things that are necessary to create my life are in me. In more than a whimsical sense, I believe that I am God and I believe that you are, and both of those statements are very important."[10]

Anyone who explores the length and breadth of the holistic movement will bump into universal energy in almost every form of alternative therapy. In many cases (such as ancient Chinese medicine) the idea is central and overt; in others (such as homeopathy) it lies beneath the surface in the theory which explains the practice. In the next few pages we will present a few examples of the universal-energy concept in diverse forms.

Prana: Energy from the Air

From ancient Hinduism comes the idea that universal energy flows from the air we breathe (hence the word *prana*, from the Sanskrit word for "breath"). The various schools of yoga place much emphasis on breathing techniques and exercises, known as pranayama, which are said to concentrate prana from the air and distribute it throughout the body. While we might tend to think of yoga as a series of exercises for improving flexibility and muscle tone, yogic practices (from whatever school) are intended to produce altered states of consciousness. (The word *yoga* comes from the Sanskrit term for "yoke" or "union," and yogic exercises are ultimately intended to produce an experience of union with Brahman, the impersonal god of Hinduism. The widespread availability of yoga classes in health clubs and physical education programs has unfortunately given these practices an air of innocence and spiritual neutrality which they scarcely deserve. One should not take yoga's mystical underpinnings and occult ties lightly.)[11]

Some might argue that the Hindu mystics simply gave oxygen a name before it was isolated scientifically. Modern mystics allow us no such conclusion. One contributor to *A Visual Encyclopedia of Unconventional Medicine* informs us that "in some areas of the world there is a high concentrtion of prana, particularly at the seaside, at high altitudes, and in an abundance of sunshine."[12] (Anyone with chronic lung disease can testify that there is no abundance of oxygen at high altitude.) Another author, Yogi Ramarcharaka, describes how one can hang on to prana if it seems to be slipping away:

> If you feel that your vital energy is at a low ebb and you need to build up and store a new supply quickly, the best plan is to place the feet close together, side by side, and lock the fingers of both hands. This closes the circuit and prevents any escape of prana through the extremities. Then breathe rhythmically a few times and you will feel the effects of the recharging.[13]

Many teachers claim that prana can be focused, using meditative techniques, at seven energy centers or vortices called *chakras*. Located in the midline of the body, the chakras are given various titles and assumed to regulate both physiological and psychic events. (Some have said that the chakras correlate with the endocrine glands, although the ancient mystics to whom we owe this system had no specific knowledge of endocrine function.)

In addition, some writers describe what is considered among psychics to be the most potent flow of energy within the body: the rising of the *kundalini*. Within the spinal column is said to exist an energy conduit; if prana is channeled through this canal, from the base of the spine to the base of the skull, one experiences the rising of the kundalini, with all powers and terrors appertaining thereto. All who describe the kundalini warn of its power to destroy as well as heal. Even under the supervision of an experienced teacher, one who manipulates this energy is considered liable to experience severe physical reactions, psychosis or even death.

The ideas of chakras and kundalini are loaded with mystical and sexual overtones. Mary Coddington describes the purpose for mastering the kundalini:

> The kundalini is a goddess as well as a snake, and she lies in three and one-half coils in her cave (kanda) at the base of the

spine. The purpose of kundalini yoga is to rouse the sleeping kundalini so that she stretches, hisses, and writhes her way up through the sushumna channel to the top of the head where the Lord Shiva, third god of the Hindu trinity, abides. Shiva represents pure consciousness, and kundalini is a power of the goddess Shakti. The aim of kundalini yoga is accomplished with the union or marriage of Shiva and Shakti.[14]

One form of yoga known as *tantra* teaches specific techniques to raise kundalini through sexual intercourse. Tantric lovers visualize currents of prana flowing through them during their meditative embrace, in which they are "using their bodies and the joined magnitude of their complementary forces as a vehicle through which to achieve the rising of the Kundalini and the awakening of spiritual consciousness."[15]

What is the ultimate goal of manipulating universal energy, according to the purveyors of prana? Learning to relax? Healing the sick? Coping with the stress of life? These may be fringe benefits, but they are child's play compared to the end point, which is to become God. Swami Vivekananda states it eloquently as he portrays the powers of the fully enlightened yogi:

> What power on earth would not be his? He would be able to move the sun and stars out of their places, to control everything in the universe from the atoms to the biggest suns. This is the end and aim of pranayama. When the yogi becomes perfect there will be nothing in nature not under his control. If he orders the gods or the souls of the departed to come, they will come at his bidding. All the forces of nature will obey him as slaves. . . . He who has controlled prana has controlled his own mind and all the minds, . . . and all the bodies that exist.[16]

Mana: The Power of the Kahuna

In Polynesian culture universal energy is called *mana* and is the force used by Polynesian shamans (known as *kahunas*) in the practice of "white" and "black" magic. As described by Max Freedom Long in *The Secret Science behind Miracles*, the kahuna traditions describe a complex spiritual anatomy, involving a separate invisible "etheric" body for each of three selves: the low, middle and high. The low self is primitive, controlling appetites and desires. It directs energy which can move physical objects. The etheric body of the low self is sticky and connects a person via invisible threads to anything else which is touched. The middle self is conscious and rational, and its etheric body is the form in which one's spirit survives after death. The higher self is a sort of resident god or guardian angel, knowing past, present and much of the future. Its etheric body uses a high-powered energy called *mana loa*, which is responsible for all miraculous events.

These three selves have an interesting communication system. The high and low selves are in touch with one another, without the middle being aware of it. Furthermore, the conscious, middle self can only appeal to the powerful, all-knowing high self by contacting the low self, which will relay the message. Mastering this inner switchboard is a goal of the budding kahuna.

While this system may sound like a mishmash of mythology and Freud, it reflects an important idea which is spreading through the holistic health movement and society at large. The residence of the middle self is said to be the left half of the brain, which many authors claim to be the center of conscious, rational, deductive thinking. The higher self, on the other hand, lives in the right half of the brain, which the same authors describe as the center of intuitive, creative thinking, the realm of the higher consciousness. One of the major themes of the New Consciousness is that Western society has developed all of its technological wizardry and problems as a result of left-brain thinking, to the exclusion of the right brain. The New Age, we are told, will see the awakening of the right brain with all of its untapped wisdom and power.

It should be noted that some fascinating research has in fact been carried out in an effort to elucidate the function and capabilities of each side of the brain. The details are too involved to discuss here, but for the interested reader we recommend D. Gareth Jones's book *Our Fragile Brains*.[17] In holistic health circles, the emphasis is almost always on the mystical and metaphysical dimensions of this idea and rarely on clinical details.

The kahuna system, which some have praised as a highly sophisticated, comprehensive metaphysical system, is also overtly spiritistic and leaves the doors of consciousness wide open for contact with nonphysical entities. Some kahunas have stated that spirits of the dead make contact with the higher self to assist in psychic feats or to manipulate mana (for good or ill) in others. To make matters more confusing, the mana energy itself is described in terms which suggest that it has its own independent intelligence.

Shamanistic world views and practices such as those of the kahunas are studied now not only by anthropologists in a purely academic light, but also by those who see them as a means for tapping supernatural powers. Indeed, early in the twentieth century observers such as William Tufts Brigham, curator of the Bishop Museum in Honolulu, described what appears to be miraculous healings, weather control, firewalking and control of animal behavior (such as calling sharks into shallow water) through exercise of the occult wisdom of the kahuna. While few organizations specifically promote the cultivation of mana, the positive attitude expressed toward shamanism in some corners of the holistic health movement is a fascinating turnabout in a technological society.

Ch'i: The Foundation of Acupuncture
The Ch'i energy concept, derived from the ancient Chinese mystical philosophy known as Taoism, is at the core of traditional acupuncture and acupressure techniques. It is also invoked to explain a variety of rather unorthodox practices which are promoted everywhere from some chiropractors' offices to *Family Circle* magazine. Ch'i is such an important idea that we will devote all of Part II to it.

Universal Energy in Action: Therapeutic Touch
The practice of Therapeutic Touch is a prime example of an ancient concept—prana—dressed in contemporary garb so as to gain wide acceptability. Its chief promoter is Dolores Krieger, R.N., Ph.D., who has taught this technique primarily to nurses. Her class at New York University, entitled "Frontiers in Nursing: The Actualization of Potential for Therapeutic Human Field Interaction," has been

attended by hundreds of nurses as part of their masters or doctoral programs. Continuing education courses nationwide have trained thousands of other health professionals in similar techniques.

In her book *The Therapeutic Touch*, Krieger describes how she became acquainted with the idea of healing through touch while studying Hungarian healer Oskar Estebany. (While a colonel in the Hungarian cavalry, Estebany had discovered by accident an ability to heal animals and humans through the laying on of hands.) Later, under the tutelage of psychic Dora Kunz, Krieger began to experiment with the transfer of human energies and eventually developed a theory for her experiences. While her academic background had been neurophysiology, her understanding of Therapeutic Touch came from the East through the study of yoga, Aruvedic (that is, Hindu) medicine and Chinese medicine. She concluded that prana—the Hindu version of universal energy—is "at the base of the human energy transfer in the healing act":

> Conceive of the healer as an individual whose health gives him access to an overabundance of prana and whose strong sense of commitment and intention to help ill people gives him or her a certain control over the projection of this vital energy. The act of healing, then, would entail the channeling of this energy flow by the healer for the well-being of the sick individual.[18]

The fact that Eastern mysticism is the cornerstone of Therapeutic Touch is made clear from the outset in Krieger's book. The idea that "prana may be transferred from one individual to another may not be so readily apparent to us unless we have gotten into the *practice* and literature of hatha yoga, tantric yoga, or the martial arts of the orient."[19]

The practitioner of Therapeutic Touch is seen not as a generator of energy, but as a conduit, one who directs energy where it is needed. Beneficial effects to the patient are said to include pain relief, generalized relaxation and an improvement of illnesses which have a significant psychological component (for example, some cases of asthma). Krieger also reports positive responses (such as improved growth and neurological development) in premature infants treated informally by nurses and parents in New York University's intensive-care nursery.

Therapeutic Touch is described as a four-step process. Step one is called *centering*, a meditative process of becoming quiet and relaxed, developing a state of inner equilibrium.

Step two is *assessment*, the scanning of the patient's energy fields with the hands. The healer places his or her hands two to three inches from the patient's body and slowly moves over both front and back surfaces. The object is to perceive subtle sensations such as temperature changes, tingling, pressure or pulsation, all of which are said to reflect variations in the energy field.

This perception, and its interpretation, are not meant to be equivalent to standard medical diagnosis; in fact, there is little or no relation between the two:

> Every facet of Therapeutic Touch is concerned with energy flow.
> . . . From this point of view, one can easily see that a medical diagnosis would be highly inappropriate, since medical diagnoses arise out of a classification system that is unlike the perceptions we are dealing with. The perceptions . . . are at a very direct, perhaps primitive level. Medical diagnosis, on the other hand, is based upon a very complex system of classification that is quite sophisticated, and so there is little relation between the two; indeed, there is little reason why there should be, or why there need be.[20]

Step three involves *unruffling the field*, the process of decongesting the energy flow. When the healer perceives a sense of pressure while scanning the body, he or she is said to be bumping against stagnant energy. The cure is to sweep the energy downward with the hands, thus paving the way for the transfer of energy in the next step.

Step four, *the transfer of energy*, moves energy from the healer to the patient or from one place to another within the body of the patient. In Krieger's approach, the healer uses the sensations felt in the hands in step two as a guide for treatment. An area which feels hot needs to be cooled, a cool area warmed, an area of tingling quieted and so forth. These changes are brought about as the healer creates the desired feeling (cool in place of warm) in his or her mind and then directs this image through the hands.

The practice of Therapeutic Touch is highly intuitive and subjective, having been aptly described as a healing meditation. It may come as no surprise, then, that changes in the thinking of the healer assume a significance as great as (if not greater than) any effects on the patient. Krieger describes two important types of changes. First, those who regularly use Therapeutic Touch may develop "natural faculties . . . which our culture allows to lie dormant within us."[21] The most common of these is telepathy—nonverbal, nonphysical communication. Krieger comments that "if the healer is trying to get in intuitive touch with another, to learn to react sensitively to that person's 'vibes,' it should not come as a surprise that he or she is going to succeed in developing latent abilities in communication."[22]

Second, Krieger writes that the process of healing through touch can and should lead to the exploration of one's unconscious mind, the "farther reaches of the psyche."[23] She recommends that her students learn to tap the subconscious by recording its symbolic expressions, which may be brought forth through various techniques. "There are several ways of doing this, but I find that the recording of dreams, the drawing of mandalas, and divination by means of consulting the I Ching most useful. . . . I find that all three . . . integrate the search for one's own authentic nature in a unitive manner which can be very creative as well as enlightening."[24]

The Medium Is the Message

Therapeutic Touch epitomizes the thrust of almost every therapy based on universal energy. A mystical concept is extracted from a distant corner of Eastern philosophy, sanitized in Western scientific trappings, and then taught to well-intentioned members of the helping professions who are looking for new ways to relieve suffering. Krieger begins by telling us that we can learn to heal, and before long she has us developing psychic communication, drawing mandalas (complex visual patterns used for meditation), and practicing an ancient form of fortunetelling. Whatever their initial appeal, energy therapies inevitably beckon the budding healer into more "hard-core" New Consciousness thinking, since these systems are in essence profoundly mystical and often occultic. The healing method and the religious message are inseparable.

Energy enthusiasts will often tie their ideas (however loosely) to the findings of the scientific establishment, but almost all of what they say arises from the combination of their world view and their personal experiences (usually involving altered states of consciousness). Their fire is fueled by a core of mystical physicists who believe they have found a unifying connection between Eastern mysticism (especially Advaita Vedantic Hinduism, Mahayana Buddhism, and Taoism) and modern quantum mechanics. (Fritjof Capra's The Tao of Physics is a notable example of this thinking.)[25]

It must be noted, however, that the current interest in universal energy is not the result of research by scores of neutral investigators in diverse fields. No one can construct an airtight proof that universal energy exists or demonstrate its effects in a reproducible experiment to unbiased observers. Instead, many believers point to specific cases of healings or to inner experiences and declare them to be the handiwork of this invisible energy.

The crucial question is not just whether objective (or subjective) healings actually take place, but what they mean. If a patient feels more relaxed after a session of Therapeutic Touch, is it because prana has been unruffled or because the healer's voice and manner were soothing? If acupuncture produces pain relief, does it mean that energy has been turned loose, or have nerve endings been stimulated to block pain messages entering the spinal cord?

Obviously, a great deal hinges on how one interprets such occurrences, and in the kingdom of universal energy all interpretation proceeds from the spiritual precepts of the New Consciousness. The New Consciousness may be boiled down to four basic ideas which form the cornerstone of most Eastern mysticism and occult metaphysics.[26]

1. "All is one." This summary statement of the world view known as monism is not a theoretical proposition, but rather a conclusion drawn from experiences in altered states of consciousness (such as those induced through taking drugs or meditating). The

individual experiences the disappearance of all distinctions between himself or herself and all other objects and individuals, as well as between good and evil, which are said to be nothing more than different sides of the same reality. One must enter an altered state to accept this, since normal consciousness does not support the idea that I am you, you are a tree, my dog is a rock and so on.

2. "Man is a divine being." If there is only one single reality, which various religions have designated as god, then we are all parts of it. Our innermost self must therefore be divine (or god), even if our behavior suggests otherwise. The most profound chasm exists here between the New Consciousness and the teachings of the Old and New Testaments. Scripture declares that God is the Creator and that human beings are the creatures; the creatures are distinct from the Creator and, among other things, are to worship God and not themselves. Whether one accepts the role of creature or assumes oneself to be God is a central issue of the Bible.

3. "The purpose of life is to become aware of our divine nature." Since we are all emanations of one reality, the New Consciousness states that there is no need for forgiveness or salvation. Instead, individuals need enlightenment to understand their own divinity. (*Illumination, self-realization, at-one-ment* are examples of terms equivalent to enlightenment.) One comes to understand the nature of divinity using various spiritual and psychic techniques.

4. "Enlightenment leads to the exercise of 'psychospiritual' power." As an individual progresses in knowledge of the reality which exists beyond our five senses, manipulations of the spiritual and physical worlds become possible by controlling one's consciousness. Matter may be created or destroyed, and the miraculous can become commonplace.

Universal energy is, indeed, a crucial link between mysticism and the everyday world, and every energy therapy comes with strings attached—strings which ultimately pull toward the world of the paranormal, toward the exaltation of self as divine, or toward overt occultism. Unfortunately, the connection may not be evident to the well-meaning therapist or to someone seeking healing. To these we reiterate an old adage: let the buyer beware.

Part II
Ancient
Chinese
Medicine

If there were an award for the best performance in a supporting role in the holistic health movement, it would undoubtedly be won by the ancient Chinese. Within one generation, the products of Chinese medicine—especially acupuncture and acupressure—have risen from utter obscurity to household familiarity in the Western world. Acupuncture has graduated from a "Ripley's Believe It or Not" curiosity to a treatment for chronic pain in prestigious university medical centers. Acupressure techniques are presented to shoppers in the magazines at supermarket check-out stands. Applied kinesiology, a unique blend of Chinese medicine and American chiropractic theory, is gaining popularity in a variety of formats. Other imports from the ancient Orient, such as T'ai Chi Ch'uan, are less familiar to the general public but commonly taught at holistic health centers.

Many Americans have stumbled across one or another form of Chinese medicine without recognizing it as such. A neighbor talks of having her energies balanced by a local therapist. A coworker describes how his chiropractor tested his muscles to find an underlying organic problem. A relative is altering her diet as a result of testing muscle strength while holding various foods in her mouth. Whether one's response is curiosity or amusement, it is important to know something about the origins of these therapies.

Why is this important? Because unknowingly Aunt Mary and Mr. Jones may be slowly conforming their beliefs to an ancient metaphysical system called Taoism as a result of their exposure to these muscle tests for food allergies and holistic chiropractic sessions. People who know nothing of ancient Chinese religion will tell how energy flows through their bodies in invisible channels. Individuals who would never dream of calling themselves Taoists are concerned about whether they have an imbalance of yin and yang. In essence, Chinese medicine is providing a way for people (including many Christians who accept Scripture as authoritative) to act like mystics without realizing it and perhaps to become mystics.

As with so many other Eastern imports (such as meditation or the martial arts), the transformation of thinking comes along with a simple technique for achieving some other purpose, such as relaxation or feeling more energetic. Overall there is a woeful lack of discernment in this area, both in the secular and the Christian world. Our first step toward filling this void will be to take a close look at the historic roots of Chinese medicine.

4
The
Mystical
Roots

THE ORIGINS OF CLASSICAL Chinese medicine are obscure, buried in thousands of years of tradition. Nevertheless, its first and most important textbook is universally recognized to be the *Huang Ti Nei Ching Su Wen,* or *The Yellow Emperor's Classic of Internal Medicine* (which we will refer to as the *Nei Ching*). Its author, the "Yellow Lord" Huang Ti, is said in some genealogies to have lived from 2697 to 2597 B.C. and reigned as the third of China's first five rulers. Actually, there is some disagreement as to whether he existed at all. Accounts of his wisdom as a ruler mingle with tales of his miraculous conception and the appearance of the phoenix at the close of his reign. Mythological or not, he has been held in high esteem and was at one time worshiped semiannually in China.[1]

The date and authorship of the *Nei Ching* are open to question, since its original contents have been thoroughly sifted by commentators over the centuries. The best edition available today dates from A.D. 762, thirty-four hundred years from the reign of Huang

Ti. In spite of such uncertainty, the Nei Ching has been, like its legendary author, the object of highest regard in Chinese medicine. It is not a textbook as such but rather a series of dialogues between Huang Ti and his minister Ch'i Po. The emperor poses questions which are promptly answered in long discourses ranging into general ethics and metaphysics. Historian Ilza Veith comments in her excellent introduction to the Nei Ching, "This combination is, as a matter of fact, the only way in which early Chinese medical thinking could be expressed, for medicine was but a part of philosophy and religion, both of which propounded oneness with nature, i.e., the universe."[2]

Veith hits the nail on the head. Chinese medicine is the child of Chinese religion, and at their core both have the same ingredients: the Tao, yin and yang, the universal energy Ch'i, and the five elements.

The Tao

The ancient Chinese produced many philosophical systems, of which two are most familiar in the West. One, Confucianism, stressed social order and practical knowledge, forming the basis for formal education and etiquette. Taoism, on the other hand, was far more mystical. Its spiritual father, Lao-tze (literally, "the old master"), expounded on the concept of the Tao, or "the way," an impersonal concept of ultimate reality.

Taoism is centered on the importance of process and change, the concept that nature and the universe flow in an endless course of continuous cycles. Day becomes night, winter turns to spring, warm things cool, wet becomes dry, and so on, all in observable patterns. Taoism urges human beings, who are seen as utterly dependent on nature, to live in harmony with these cycles and thus to be "one" with the Tao. The person who does so is promised success and long life, while the person who "bucks the system" of nature will suffer failure, disease and an early grave.

Yin and Yang

Yin and yang are said to be the two fundamental forces which generate all of the transformations in the universe. These forces are bi-*polar,* meaning that they are opposites which are not antagonistic. They do not cancel each other, but are part of the same whole, much as the North and South Poles are opposite ends of the same planet. The words *yin* and *yang* literally mean "the shady and sunny sides of a hill," but they have come to encompass a wealth of character-istics (see table below).

Yin		Yang	
dark	yielding	light	firm
moon	west/north	sun	east/south
night	metal	day	wood
cold	white/black	heat	green/red
water	rest	fire	movement
dampness	spring/summer	dryness	autumn/winter
feminine (wife)	interior	masculine (husband)	exterior
below	contraction	above	expansion

All events in nature and in human lives are said to be influenced by the ever-changing interplay of these forces. Neither is said to exist in an absolute state, but small amounts of each are contained in the other, as illustrated by the familiar ancient symbol *T'ai-chi T'u,* the "Diagram of the Supreme Ultimate."

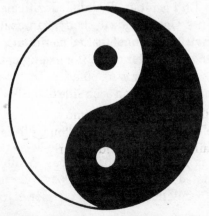

This figure has been impressed into popular consciousness over the past several years, decorating a large variety of objects from T-shirts to calendars.

Although yang sometimes is given virtuous characteristics (life, nobility, beauty) and yin correspondingly negative values (death, commonness, ugliness), they are not considered good and evil principles, but only complementary attributes of the same reality. (Likewise, what appears to be good and evil on earth are, in fact, only contrasting aspects of the same unity. The Taoist sage, in theory, sees beyond good and evil.)

The *Nei Ching* applies the interaction of yin and yang to the human body in excruciating detail. The inside of the body is yin, the surface yang, the front yin and the back yang. Each major organ of the body is designated as either yin or yang, depending on which force dominates its function. The entire body is divided into lower, middle and upper regions, each of which has yin and yang subdivisions, which in turn have two specific organs. Health is then defined as the state in which yin and yang are in perfect, dynamic balance over a period of time, with disease occurring when there is an excess of yin or yang accumulating anywhere in the body.

Ch'i

The key (no pun intended) to Chinese medicine lies in this concept of universal, invisible life energy which is said to flow through all living organisms. *Ch'i* is reputedly inhaled with air and extracted from food and drink. Once inside the body, it finds its way to a network of twelve invisible channels called *meridians,* each of which is associated with a particular organ (for example, heart, bladder) and shares that organ's yin or yang polarity. The twelve meridians are duplicated symmetrically on each side of the body and divided into closely associated pairs.

The *Nei Ching* teaches that in health Ch'i flows freely through the meridians in a one-way circuit which vaguely resembles a road with hairpin turns at the fingertips and toes. While ten of the meridians are associated with known organs, two are named for nonexistent organs: Circulation and Triple Warmer. Various vague explanations for these are given in modern acupuncture literature.

Illness, as stated previously, occurs when the flow of Ch'i through the body is obstructed or excessive in any area, thus disrupting the balance of yin and yang. Healing occurs when balance is restored.

In the *Nei Ching* specific diseases, such as pneumonia or diabetes, did not exist. Instead, imbalances of yin and yang were referred to by names such as "injuries of the heart," "injuries of the stomach" and so on. Certain forms of fever were also recognized. (Modern acupuncturists often claim to cure an impressive roster of diseases, whose names are generally supplied by Western medicine. Nevertheless, there is a tendency in modern acupuncture textbooks to describe treatments for catchall diagnoses such as "heart problems" or "prostate trouble.")

Diagnosis

In diagnosing the cause of an illness, the patient's complaints, overall appearance, color and breathing pattern are taken into account, but according to the *Nei Ching* the key to correct diagnosis is examination of the pulses. At each wrist the radial pulse (the one on the thumb side) is divided (according to the *Nei Ching*) into three zones, each of which has a superficial and deep position. These

The Twelve Pulses of Ancient Chinese Medicine

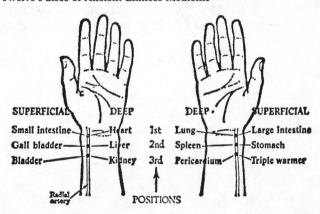

twelve pulse locations correspond to the twelve meridians and are said to communicate to the examiner information about the meridians. Each pulse position (shown in the diagram) is carefully felt and the pulse characterized using any of several adjectives, such as full, weak, floating, slippery or wiry. Pulses are interpreted in light of several factors, including time of day, season of the year and sex of the patient (with a woman's right pulse to be examined first, a man's left). Incidentally, no acupuncture textbook explains what to do for an amputee.

This diagnostic process may require thirty minutes or more, but the Chinese physician is said to be rewarded with knowledge of imbalances in any given organ, a precise diagnosis and even prognostic information, including warnings of unsuspected disease. This miraculous ability of the radial pulses to communicate information about the entire body would seem to require a clairvoyant examiner. It has no basis in physiology.

Treatment

Once the physician has made the appropriate diagnosis, the Nei Ching offers five basic approaches to therapy. The first is treatment of the spirit, guiding the patient toward the Tao in the practice of a modest, tranquil way of life. The second and third are dietary and medicinal therapies, the fourth treatment is acupuncture (or one of its variants), and the fifth is massage. Overall, the ancient text devotes relatively few pages to therapy as compared to diagnosis. It was apparently assumed that the physician knew what to do once the problem was identified.

Of the five therapies, the Nei Ching gives the most attention to acupuncture, but without any basic instructions. The origin of this method is totally unknown, although one author suggests that cold weather forced the earliest physicians to develop a method of treatment which would not require removing the patient's clothes.[3] Others have suggested that the ancients noticed distant reactions to local injury and slowly accumulated their observations, over hundreds of years, into a system of therapy. Whatever their origin, the techniques of acupuncture were refined over the centuries and eventually spread to other Asian countries. During the seventeenth century they were introduced in Europe.

Needles of all shapes and sizes have been used, some rather terrifying in appearance. At the present time most therapists use stainless-steel needles ranging in length from one-half to four inches. When points of insertion are selected, one or more needles are inserted and advanced until a sensation described as "tingling, distention, heaviness, and numbness" is felt by the patient.[4] The needles are then twisted manually or connected to an electrical pulse generator for ten to fifteen minutes. (The electrical approach has become increasingly popular, since less effort is required of the therapist.)

Alternately, points may be injected with water, saline, lidocaine, vitamin B-12 or virtually any other sterile substance. Sometimes a catgut thread is inserted at one point, pulled out at another, and left in place for days or weeks for long-term stimulation. A traditional variant is the practice of moxibustion, in which a smoldering fragment of the plant Artimisia Vulgaris is placed on or near the acupuncture point.

For the faint-hearted patient who would prefer not to be punctured, injected or burned, simple finger pressure may be used. Many variants of this technique, referred to as acupressure, are popular and widely used today. More creative therapists zap points with laser beams or buzz them with ultrasound.

In classical acupuncture therapy, the goal is to correct imbalances of yin and yang by stimulating specific points along the twelve meridians, thereby draining excesses of energy or restoring deficiencies. Various authors recognize anywhere from 365 to 800 points, the lower number being more widely accepted. These are mapped on charts and mannequins, and located on the patient using landmarks of surface anatomy. The guidelines for selecting acupuncture points have evolved into a system which is too complex for all but the most dedicated therapist. The underlying principles are contained in the "Law of the Five Elements," a concept which, like yin, yang, Ch'i and pulse diagnosis, seems grounded in mysticism.

The Five Elements

The ancient Chinese conceived of everything in the world as belonging to one of five categories: wood, fire, earth, metal and water. These were thought to represent tangible components, or "creations," of yin and yang. They are vaguely similar to the discredited Western idea that all matter consists of earth, air, fire and water. The Chinese system is more complex, in that the five elements interact with one another in a specific manner. Each "creates" another (for example, wood creates fire) and is "subjugated" by a third (for example, metal subjugates wood). In addition, each of the five elements is associated with a particular color, season, direction, flavor (the basis of dietary therapies), odor, sound and musical note; and each organ in the human body is related to one of the elements.

The overall system is often represented by a diagram of interconnected circles. This diagram, which is reproduced in nearly all traditional acupuncture textbooks, is a roadmap of sorts for routing energies, since surplus Ch'i is said to travel only in the direction shown by the arrows. Memorizing the map is felt to be essential to the classical therapist. One textbook, *Acupuncture Therapy* by Mary Austin, gives examples such as the following of a diagnosis and its corresponding treatment:

The pulse diagnosis indicates:

DEFICIENCY ON XII (Spleen)   Earth organ
EXCESS ON IX (Lungs)   Metal organ

First, we draw upon Wood by the control device of supplementing the wood point on the spleen meridian. This starts an energy movement by drawing on the normal towards the deficiency—thus creating a small deficiency on the Wood organ VIII (liver). We now can act upon this artificially created deficiency to draw the surplus from the Metal by supplementing at the metal point on the liver meridian. This treatment involves action at two points.[5]

In addition to this, the season of the year, phase of the moon, weath-

The Five Elements and Their Relationships

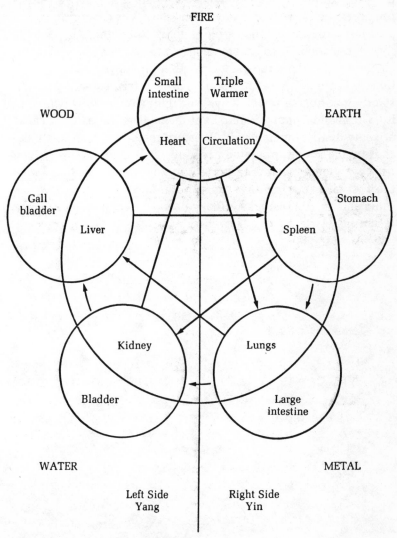

Outer Arrows: "Creating" relationships
Inner Arrows (star pattern): "Subjugating" relationships

er and time of day all affect the flow of yin and yang and thus the choice of points and needling techniques. Even the choice of flavors in the patient's diet, because of their tie to the five elements, has to be carefully considered. One wonders if someday an enterprising therapist will take away the guesswork by designing an acupuncture program for the Apple II home computer.

Without probing any more deeply into ancient Chinese medicine, it is clear that this system is both highly mystical in orientation and seemingly incongruous with Western science's understanding of human physiology. We might wonder why people in industrialized America would be attracted to it. Yet partly because of some disillusionment with Western medicine, and partly because of the scientific community's interest in acupuncture (which has contributed an air of respectability), we are seeing this Taoist offshoot take root in American culture. To understand how this came about, we must take a look at some of acupuncture's more recent history.

5
Acupuncture's Questionable Triumphs

TRADITIONAL PRACTICES BASED on the *Nei Ching* were the only treatments available in China until the nineteenth century, when cross-fertilization from Europe introduced Western concepts of healing to the Orient. As unrefined as these were, they were convincing enough to bring about an order for the abandonment of acupuncture by the Great Imperial Medical Board in 1822 and again by the Kuomintang government in 1929. Nevertheless, the old practices survived, partly because of resistance to change among the large rural population. More importantly, there was a great scarcity of Western-trained physicians. Only 20,000 to 30,000 of these were in practice, mostly in urban centers, when Mao Tse-tung came to power in 1949. The remaining eighty per cent of China's 550,000,000 population was served by roughly 40,000 traditional physicians.

The sweeping social changes brought about by the Communist regime included reorganization of the entire medical system, with a concurrent revival of interest in the traditional methods. Playing to the preference of the rural population, Chairman Mao stressed the virtue of traditional medicine in pronouncements such as: "Chinese medicine and pharmacology are a great treasure house; efforts should be made to explore them and raise them to higher levels."[1]

The process of integrating Chinese and Western medicine was accelerated by the onslaught of the Great Proletariat Cultural Revolution in 1966. During this frantic social upheaval, universities and medical schools were closed, college students and professors were shipped to the countryside for "re-education," and publication of scientific journals ground to a halt. The only technical skill recognized to be of any value was the fervent recitation of the "Sayings of Chairman Mao."

When the dust finally settled, medical schools were reopened with a curriculum cut from six years to three, an emphasis on practical training in the countryside, and an invigorated study of traditional medicine. The latter was given equal billing with Western medicine. It came to be studied in greater detail by scientific researchers and was practiced in hospitals side by side with Western methods. Patients now could choose which approach they preferred, with traditional medicine especially strong in the countryside, where "barefoot doctors" (farmers who were trained in basic first aid) acted as the initial medical contact for most of the population.

Fascinated Westerners
These developments created less than a ripple of interest in the West until 1971, when James Reston, an editorial columnist and vice president of the *New York Times*, became one of the first American reporters in years to visit mainland China. Reston viewed a number of surgical operations, including the removal of a tuberculous lung and the excision of a brain tumor, in which the patient remained awake and alert—with acupuncture apparently the sole anesthetic. During his visit to Peking, Reston suffered an attack of appendicitis, requiring surgery for which a spinal anesthetic was used. Postoperatively he developed stomach cramps, which were

diagnosed as gastritis and treated successfully by an acupuncturist. Reston's report of these episodes in the *New York Times* (22 August 1971) and in media interviews stirred widespread interest.

Within the next several months journalists, scientists and physicians made pilgrimages to China, most reporting their observations in the popular press and a few in scientific journals. (President Nixon's personal physician, Dr. Walter Tkach, for example, wrote his summary in *Today's Health,* while cardiologist E. Grey Dimond published a series of articles for the *Journal of the American Medical Association.*) The articles reported that thousands of successful operations of all kinds were being carried out in China using acupuncture anesthesia: craniotomies (opening the skull), thyroid surgery, tonsillectomies, Cesarean sections, and even lung and open-heart surgeries. Dr. Tkach was so impressed that he declared that the Chinese "have something very superior to our own method of anesthesia."[2] Superior or not, the apparent success of acupuncture threw a monkey wrench into time-honored theories of the mechanism and control of pain.

Other stories described the Chinese use of acupuncture for a host of pain problems, both short-term and chronic, and some claimed miraculous cures for paralysis and deafness. Americans began to read that Winston Churchill, John F. Kennedy, Willie McCovey of the San Francisco Giants, Prince Bernhard of the Netherlands and Roman Gabriel of the Los Angeles Rams had all received acupuncture treatments for control of pain. By early 1972 a boom of sorts had started, as practitioners possessing varying amounts of education and scruples began to treat an ever-enlarging clientele. Those with aspirations in business began sponsoring correspondence courses and seminars, distributing do-it-yourself acupuncture paraphernalia, and opening Chinese medicine clinics. The needles eventually found their way into university medical centers (especially those with pain clinics), as well as some private physicians' offices. More recently, courses in acupressure and other derivatives of classical Chinese medicine (such as *Jin Shin Do, Tai Chi Ch'uan* and especially Touch for Health) became widely available.

As the scientific community began to take a harder look at the acupuncture phenomenon, some questions were raised which had escaped notice of the popular press. Does Chinese medicine work as advertised? How successful is it, especially when compared to other forms of treatment (or no treatment at all)? Are its effects influenced by such variables as the type of disease, the prevalent beliefs in the culture, or the emotional make-up of the patient? Are the specific points used or the type of stimulation really important? If acupuncture works in a significant number of cases, by what mechanism? Could these practices be used with any success in the West?

These questions are not the academic quibblings of the ivory tower set, but questions which must be asked of any therapy, whether a sophisticated new antibiotic or Dr. Wonder's Snake Oil. One or even many personal experiences do not establish the validity of any therapy, although they may stimulate interest or demand an explanation. While many people couldn't care less what science thinks of Chinese medicine as long as it works for them, for others the endorsement of the scientific community is a crucial factor in their belief level and willingness to try something new and unusual.

What kind of evidence does ancient Chinese medicine have going for it?

Does Acupuncture Work?

It would seem, from the initial reports written by Western observers in China, that the answer is a clear-cut yes, especially in the area of pain reduction. Unfortunately, many of these travelers, even those with medical degrees, lacked the experience necessary to evaluate what they were shown.

Some especially interesting commentary was written by Dr. John J. Bonica, chairman of both the department of anesthesiology at the University of Washington and the Ad Hoc Committee of Acupuncture of the National Institutes of Health, and a long-time student of the phonomenon of pain. Bonica's careful observations of acupuncture anesthesia in China illuminated a number of facts which were misunderstood by previous observers.

Initial reports, for example, suggested that this form of anesthesia was used in the majority of surgical operations in China. From statistics supplied by the Chinese, however, Bonica calculated that it is used in less than ten per cent of all cases. Furthermore, while apparently reducing the sensation of pain, acupuncture usually does not totally eliminate pain or other uncomfortable sensations. (Some writers have observed that the word *anesthesia*, meaning "absense of sensation," does not apply to acupuncture, and that the word *hypalgesia*, meaning "decrease of pain," is more appropriate.)

Nearly every patient receives, in addition to needling, a narcotic or barbiturate injection prior to surgery or a slow "drip" of narcotic (usually Demerol) into a vein during the operation. Local anesthesia is frequently injected into sensitive structures before they are cut or manipulated. Acupuncture does not produce muscle relaxation, making some abdominal operations nearly impossible (tight abdominal muscles are a formidable barrier), and the unavoidable traction on internal organs may produce nausea and vomiting. To minimize this, Chinese surgeons often work with extreme deliberation when acupuncture is the main pain reliever. Emergency surgery is essentially never done using acupuncture. While in a large series of operations a ninety-four per cent rate of effectiveness was reported in a major Chinese publication, Bonica pointed out that a large number of these patients experienced pain to the point where significant supplemental medication was required. Only those who were totally unable to "grin and bear it" were included in the other six per cent.

Even with these limitations, however, it cannot be denied that a large variety (if not number) of operations has been carried out with patients awake and alert, a definite advantage in some procedures. (For example, in thyroid surgery if the patient's voice remains normal, it indicates that a nerve to the larynx has not been accidentally cut.) Other advantages of acupuncture include minimal risk, essentially no change in normal physiology (with no recovery period from anesthesia needed), simplicity, and lack of expense. No one has seriously suggested that such operations were faked.

Other applications of acupuncture in China have been widely publicized. Bonica reported claims of excellent response in many chronic pain disorders, except for pain following herpes zoster (shingles) outbreaks, chronic pain caused by advanced cancer, and emergency situations in which the patient is apprehensive. Disorders such as nerve deafness and paralysis in children following polio infections have been said to respond dramatically to acupuncture. Such claims have been recounted by Western authors whose enthusiasm often exceeded their critical judgment. Marc Duke's book Acupuncture, for example, begins with an account of one hundred fifty-one paraplegics "who had been pronounced incurable by western doctors" but were treated with acupuncture.

> Soon, some were able to wiggle their toes and feet, then bend their knees, and finally move their entire legs. They exercised for hours each day, rebuilding wasted muscles and gaining back the confidence lost in years of paralysis.

> Thirty-six months after the acupuncture treatment started, 124 or the 151 patients were able to walk without the aid of another person.[3]

These startling cures are said to be documented in Soviet and French medical journals. Unfortunately, most of the details are missing in Duke's account. In cases of hearing loss, evaluation of the cause appeared to be inadequate. Furthermore, in addition to needling points around the ears, face and limbs, extensive speech therapy was given to patients by dedicated and energetic teachers. Likewise, the intensive physical therapy given to paralysis victims, as well as some rather loose criteria for success, raise some doubts as to the role of acupuncture in reversing the ravages of polio. Bonica writes:

> Thus, any patient who can walk with assistance and has some degree of sphincter control is classified as a success regardless of the presence of any other residual neurologic disability. On the basis of these criteria it is claimed that acupuncture therapy is 95% successful in paraplegia and other serious neurologic disorders. However, it appears that the improvement in most cases

is no greater than could be expected with the use of orthodox techniques of physiotherapy and rehabilitation.[4]

Bonica's overall assessment of claims made for acupuncture, outside of the realm of pain control, was not enthusiastic:

> As far as I have been able to ascertain from my observations, discussions, and from reviews of the literature, *the claims for the high degree of efficacy of acupuncture are not based on data derived from well-controlled clinical trials.* In fact, in many health stations and even in some hospitals, no records are kept of either the patient's history or of his response to therapy. In some instances, the practitioner administrating the acupuncture could not recount for us the number of treatments and the results obtained with each treatment, simply because he did not have records.[5]

Bonica noted that many traditional therapists in China were unaware of the concept of controlled trials, where a comparison is made between patients treated with and without acupuncture. Those who were familiar with the concept felt that it would be unethical to deprive some patients of what they considered a proven form of therapy.

Conclusions similar to Bonica's regarding the use of acupuncture for surgical procedures were published in 1976 by the Acupuncture Anesthesia Study Group of the National Academy of Sciences. The twelve-member group carefully observed forty-eight operations in sixteen Chinese hospitals in May 1974. Their report echoes Bonica's observations that the degree of pain control was not as impressive as initial reports had suggested, and that certain procedures (such as thyroid operations) fared better using acupuncture than others (for example, abdominal surgery). In general, formal reports such as these, as well as the earlier summary of the NIH Ad Hoc Advisory Committee on Acupuncture in 1973, concluded that acupuncture appeared to have promise as a treatment for pain control, but that well-designed and controlled studies were necessary before advocating widespread use in the United States.

Over the years an increasing number of articles have appeared in

America and European medical journals describing the effects of acupuncture in various diseases, as well as in experimentally induced pain. In general, results have been confusing and often contradictory.[6] There has been such a lack of uniformity in the design of these experiments that conclusions can only be tentative at best. Nevertheless, the following observations may be made.

First, acupuncture does indeed relieve pain to varying degrees in a large number of patients with a wide variety of disorders, as well as during certain surgical procedures. This may seem to be stating the obvious, but there are those who still feel that the phenomenon is entirely psychological—a ritualized sugar pill.

Second, doctors cannot easily predict which patients will respond most favorably. For example, pain from terminal cancer or in emergency situations does not usually improve with acupuncture therapy. Dental pain, on the other hand, tends to respond more consistently. Cultural conditioning, belief that the procedure will work, friendly surroundings, and mood also appear to affect the results.

Third, significant pain reduction is frequently obtained by stimulating an area far removed from the location of discomfort.

Finally, the duration of pain relief may range from transient to permanent.

How Does It Work?

The results observed with acupuncture therapy serve to demonstrate that the entire phenomenon of pain is much more complex than imagined a generation ago. The old concept of "specificity"—that painful sensations from any location in the body are transmitted by a direct connection to the brain—seems appropriate when one stubs a toe, but is totally inadequate when faced with the products of Chinese medicine. Actually, many of the characteristics of acupuncture have been observed in Western medical literature, but given different names.

For example, it has been long observed that intense stimulation of one part of the body seems to decrease the sensation felt in another. This concept of *counterirritation* is an extremely old method of pain control and has been verified experimentally. (Application of a painfully cold stimulus to the leg, for example, has been found to decrease perception of pain produced by electrical stimulation of the teeth.)

The phenomenon of *referred pain*, in which pain is experienced in a location removed from the site of injury, has likewise been known to physicians for generations. The most familiar example is that of pain arising from the heart which is felt in the left shoulder or arm.

Furthermore, the existence of *trigger points* was first described by Dr. Janet Travell in 1952 and later used in the treatment of President John F. Kennedy's recurrent back trouble. Trigger points are small areas of marked local tenderness, seen usually with muscle or joint pain, which may lie in an area of referred pain or even at some distance from the problem area. It is well known that stimulating of trigger points, and especially injecting them with local anesthetic, can bring about profound and prolonged pain relief. In one review article, Dr. Ronald Melzack of McGill University, a prominent pain theorist, found a close correlation (over seventy per cent) between trigger points and acupuncture points based on both spatial relation and pain pattern.[7]

One might argue that Chinese medicine provides the explanation for these mysterious phenomena and that using a phrase such as *trigger point* is merely a convenient way for Western physicians to avoid facing the realities of meridians and Ch'i. Nevertheless, a satisfactory explanation of these observations, based on known neurological pathways without invoking universal energy, is possible within the framework of the "gate control" theory of pain described by Canadian researchers Ronald Melzack and P. D. Wall.

This concept, which has gained widespread acceptance, proposes that the transmission of pain sensations to the brain does not occur as a simple, direct connection, as when one dials a long distance phone call. Rather, many factors may alter the painful sensation before it reaches the brain, which may also alter its perception of the painful input. Melzack and Wall have proposed that a gate-like mechanism exists in the central nervous system which may be opened or closed by varying amounts such that, under certain circumstances, signals from injured tissue may not reach the brain. The gate may be closed in several ways.[8]

One way to block pain is to stimulate individual nerve fibers. Sensations from the body's surface travel through both large and small nerve fibers, with the smaller fibers transmitting most of the message of pain. Stimulating the large fibers may "close the gate" to messages from small fibers in the same nerve (or other nerves which enter the spinal cord at the same location).

The brainstem may also act as a gate, transmitting or blocking messages on their way to higher centers of the brain. Electrical stimulation of these areas in rats have been found to produce prolonged and widespread (up to half of the body) resistance to pain. This might explain why needling areas far removed from the source of pain could have definite and long-lasting effects.

The cortex of the brain—the center for memories, emotions and all higher thought processes—may also close the gate. Anxiety and fear are known to enhance the feeling of pain, as anyone who has observed childbirth can confirm. The well-trained, relaxed woman in labor will manage infinitely better than one who is frightened and unprepared. This ties in to the role of such intangible factors as the belief system of the patient, cultural experiences and faith in the therapist. This also relates to the age-old placebo effect, in which an inert substance (such as a sugar pill or a saline injection) relieves pain in a surprising number of cases (as much as thirty per cent). In general, the more convincing the suggestion that a procedure will improve pain, the more likely it is to do so.

The gate theory has been supported by the success of other kinds of local stimulation which relieve pain. One popular treatment for aching backs and sore necks is the transcutaneous nerve stimulator (TCNS), consisting of one or more pads applied to the skin and connected to a low-voltage electrical pulse generator. Many chronic pain patients carry a portable TCNS unit on their belts for continuous stimulation and long-term relief.

A newer area of pain research, which has bearing on acupuncture, suggests that an internally produced morphinelike substance (endorphins) may be secreted under a variety of conditions, perhaps including needling. The way acupuncture works (with a gradual rise in the pain threshold when needling begins and a gradual decrease when stopped) supports this hypothesis, as does the reported reversal of acupuncture analgesia by the drug naloxone. (This medication blocks the actions of opiates such as morphine and is used to reverse the effects of narcotic overdoses.)

Meridians and Ch'i: Are They Real?

We have gone to some lengths to show that the effects of acupuncture can be explained without invoking meridians and Ch'i. Unfortunately, ideas such as neurological gates and brainstem inhibition of pain do not fire the popular imagination the way universal life energy does. Furthermore, Chinese medicine and its offshoots claim to cure everything from heartburn to hemorrhoids using some type of local stimulation. Western researchers, with their primary focus on pain mechanisms, have generally ignored other medical problems, leaving a great vacuum in knowledge which energy therapists have been anxious to fill.

Before exploring the colorful world of these therapies, however, we should address a crucial question: Is there any evidence that meridians, Ch'i, yin and yang, and specific acupuncture points actually exist?

Acupuncture and acupressure enthusiasts generally adopt one of two approaches to this question. Some claim that the successes of Chinese medicine and their roster of satisfied customers validate the entire system without further proof. If it works (or seems to), nothing else matters, including an explanation. This approach seems innocuous enough. One need not understand electronics to enjoy stereo equipment, nor have mastered auto mechanics to drive the family car. Billions of aspirin tablets were consumed before anyone understood how aspirin worked.

Unfortunately, this logic does not hold water. The workings of automobiles and stereo sound may be mastered by anyone with ordinary intelligence, given enough time and some straightforward instruction. Likewise, the mechanism by which aspirin relieves headaches was unraveled using straightforward logic and experimentation. No one has swallowed a Bufferin assuming that it contained vital life forces or friendly spirits. Classical Chinese medicine stands in sharp contrast, in that the observations of the ancients—that pricking the skin in certain areas had specific results —were incorporated into the prevalent religious thinking of that era. (If similar thinking had been applied in Western culture, we might find ourselves hearing that Contac contains angels who dry the nose or Tylenol exorcises pain demons.) Not only does classical acupuncture come with its metaphysical baggage intact, but its promoters actively proclaim its religious foundations and implications as well.

Most who believe in the classical explanation of acupuncture take a second approach, that of seeking external validation. They are enthusiastic about any research which appears to support their view, and they tend to assume that such proof is at hand. John Thie, for example, makes an authoritative statement at the beginning of his *Touch for Health* handbook: "Acupressure vessels, or meridians, are located throughout the body. They contain a free-flowing, colorless, non-cellular liquid which may be partly actuated by the heart. These meridians have been measured and mapped by modern technological methods, electronically, thermaticly [sic], and radioactively."[9] One might assume from this assertion that meridians are as well defined as California's earthquake faults, but this is not the case.

The supporting research falls into three basic areas. Most of this research has been carried out in Communist countries.

The Bong Han Corpuscles
Professor Kim Bong Han of North Korea did extensive work with animals and humans which reportedly showed systems of ducts and superficial corpuscles in the skin corresponding to acupuncture points and meridians. Radioactive phosphorus (P^{32}) injected into the points of the abdominal wall of a rabbit was found to disperse along lines toward neighboring points in a manner suggesting a meridian system. (How rabbit points were determined in the first

place is not explained.) In other anatomical and histological (that is, microscopic tissue) studies, he claims to have found four systems of ducts and to have determined the electrical, mechanical, biochemical and embryological characteristics of them and the fluid they contain. (Probably this is the basis for Dr. Thie's confident statement about meridians.)

Unfortunately, none of these results have been replicated in the West, although one might argue that few scientists have been searching for Bong Han Corpuscles. It seems unlikely, however, that such an elaborate system would have escaped the notice of Western anatomists over the past five centuries. Felix Mann, an experienced English acupuncturist, cites evidence that the Bong Han structures are based on distortions of tissue occurring in the preparation of microscope slides.[10] Even if the Bong Han system is eventually verified, it remains in the realm of physical structure and offers no support for the circulation of invisible life energies.

Skin Resistance

Soviet physicist Victor Adamenko, who has actively pursued psychic research in the U.S.S.R., and surgeon Mikhail Gaikin have both used a device called a tobiscope to measure electrical resistance of skin at precise points. They have reported significant drops in resistance at locations corresponding to acupuncture points. Resistance was found to decrease even further during emotional stress, and impressive variations were measured during hypnosis. Researcher Thelma Moss, known for her extensive work in Kirlian photography (see page 76), mapped points using a similar device and found a large number which did not correlate with classical Chinese charts. Some have surmised that the tobiscope actually locates collections of sweat glands in the skin. Indeed, the measurable drop in skin resistance under emotional stress is the basis for the well-known lie detector test and has been used in psychological experimentation for years.

Felix Mann, mentioned above, through his long and successful experience with acupuncture, came to abandon the traditional theories. He now postulates that complex interactions between skin, muscle and internal organs, all mediated by the nervous system, are responsible for the effects of needling. His comments regarding skin resistance are of interest:

> Some researchers claim there is a reduced electrical skin resistance at small discrete places they call acupuncture points. For several years I have diligently tried to confirm this observation in both patients and cadavers. I found there are thousands of smaller or larger areas of reduced resistance, some of which might correspond to acupuncture points, while most did not. ...

> Each time an active electrode is passed over the skin its electrical resistance is reduced, and if this is repeated a few times one creates, de novo, one's own electrical acupuncture point.[11]

Kirlian Photography

This fascinating process, developed in the 1940s by Russian researchers Semyon and Valentina Kirlian, is frequently invoked as the final proof of universal energy, psychic healing and other assorted paranormal phenomena. To make a Kirlian photograph, a standard photographic plate is sandwiched between a high-voltage generator and an object such as a volunteer's hand or a leaf. After one or two seconds of exposure using a minuscule flow of current (to prevent burning the volunteer), the picture is developed. Typical Kirlian photos show eerie, luminous streams emanating like tiny fireworks from the surface of the object. In humans these flares have been found to change in size and intensity depending upon the volunteer's frame of mind. Skeptics consider the process to be little more than a spectacular way to record physiological changes in the skin (such as variations in moisture, temperature or electrical conductivity). Kirlian enthusiasts, however, claim that they can predict disease and prove the existence of life energies.

Sheila Ostrander and Lynn Schroeder, in their lively book *Psychic Discoveries behind the Iron Curtain*, describe how Mikhail Gaikin became interested in both acupuncture and Kirlian photography. After viewing the multicolored patterns of light seen when a human hand is photographed by the Kirlian process, Gaikin sensed a possible connection with Chinese medicine.

In the Kirlians' tiny room, as Gaikin stared at the pictures of a
human being under high-frequency fields, it seemed his hunch
had paid off. The spots where lights flared most brilliantly appeared to match the acupuncture points the Chinese had mapped
out thousands of years ago! Just possibly the Kirlian discovery
might give the first scientific confirmation of this five thousand-
year-old system of medicine. Maybe there was also a relation
between the channels of swimming light the Kirlians saw and
the pathways of Vital Energy described by the ancient Chinese.[12]
Ostrander and Schroeder extend these conjectures to develop some
far-reaching metaphysical conclusions, tying together Kirlian photography and vital energy. The authors conclude:

> Acupuncture lit up by Kirlian photography may lead to new
> forms of medical treatment, but there is a larger, perhaps ulti-
> mately more beneficial, implication in this mating of the ancient
> and the modern: a more unified view of man. This is a view of
> the human being linked to the cosmos; a view of man aware of
> and reacting, via his secondary or bioplasmic body, to changes
> in the planets, environments, and weather, as well as to ill-
> nesses, moods, and the thoughts of others; a view of man as an
> enmeshed integral part of life on earth and in the universe.[13]

This conclusion seems somewhat less likely when one examines a
few Kirlian photographs of hands and fingers. There are, in fact,
so many individual streams of light emanating from a single finger
that one would be hard pressed to identify which one corresponds
to an acupuncture point.

In the United States, many Kirlian experiments were conducted
at UCLA in the early 1970s by medical psychologist and paranormal researcher Thelma Moss. In one study, Moss stimulated a point
located (according to acupuncture charts) on the large-intestine
meridian. She simultaneously took a Kirlian photograph of the
finger tips which showed a conspicuous red spot at the theoretical
turning point of the same meridian.

The assumption is, of course, that the Kirlian photograph is doc-
umenting the invisible flow of energy between those two points.
However, the basic facts of the experiment do not necessarily de-

mand that interpretation. Moss reveals such a strong belief in the psychic realm and invisible energy flows in her book *The Probability of the Impossible* that one has to wonder whether she is imposing her own supernatural presuppositions on the results.[14]

In summary, the objective evidence that Ch'i and meridians are a part of normal human physiology is tentative, to say the least. This is not to say that nothing happens physiologically when needles are inserted into the skin or that all effects observed during acupuncture treatments are imaginary. Probably the most reasonable viewpoint is taken by British acupuncturist Felix Mann, who, as mentioned previously, postulates that the effects of acupuncture are mediated through complex neurological pathways. Mann does not believe in the existence of physical acupuncture points. His views on meridians are similar: "The meridians of acupuncture might even be compared to the meridians of geography: imaginary but useful. I hope that the investigations of neurophysiologists and others will map out the true neural pathways involved, which would then only partially correspond to meridians."[15] Of the Law of the Five Elements Mann says:

> The law of the five elements demonstrates some connections between organs well known to physiology, and some connections which presumably exist but are not yet known. In clinical practice one finds that certain of the connections happen frequently, while the others occur rarely or never. The frequently occurring connections can in most instances be more easily explained in Western terms than via the Chinese pentagram.[16]

It is clear that the Western scientific community is not rewriting all of its textbooks on the basis of its experience with Chinese medicine. The flow of Ch'i through meridians is not being taught alongside the flow of blood through the arteries and veins. Nevertheless, the effects of acupuncture on pain are playing a role in redefining our understanding of the nervous system, and experimental work continues in many centers. Whether or not Chinese medicine receives widespread acceptance by Western science as a result of controlled studies remains to be seen. The real action, however, is not in the laboratory, but in the marketplace.

6
The Popular Therapies

WHILE MOST PEOPLE in the Far East have grown up accepting acupuncture techniques, in American culture the idea of having one's skin pierced by cold steel is not greeted with enthusiasm. Responses to injections in any doctor's office vary from the grim to the hysterical, since most of us see a needle as a grotesque invader of our sacred borders. It should come as no surprise, then, that Chinese medicine packaged without needles would gain ground which acupuncture could never penetrate (so to speak). Furthermore, since anything which is quick and easy has immediate appeal, techniques which give fast results without much training could also expect a warm welcome.

The past decade has thus seen an expanding interest in therapies derived from Chinese tradition which are billed as painless, simple and quick to yield results. They are said to be a preventive, natural and holistic means of tapping our own resources to obtain optimal health. Most can be self-taught and some self-administered and are thus inexpensive. They have one additional feature, however. They are all firmly based on the mystical principles of the Nei Ching and thus are slowly infusing Taoist metaphysics into the mainstream of American culture.

Applied Kinesiology and Touch for Health

One interesting phenomenon has been the blending of the uniquely American invention, chiropractic, with the techniques of the ancient Chinese, producing an entirely new discipline with some interesting variations. Chiropractic was developed during the late 1800s by magnetic healer D. D. Palmer, who had come to the conclusion that most (if not all) bodily ailments arose from deficiencies in the transmission of vital nerve energy from the spinal cord. These blockages were said to occur because of misalignments, or subluxations, of the vertebral column, and could be corrected by appropriate manipulations. While most people today think of chiropractors primarily as physical therapists who help iron out muscular or skeletal aches and pains, in theory (and in the case of some chiropractors, in practice) spinal manipulations are supposed to help other problems as well, such as diabetes or high blood pressure. (This has led to certain conflicts with the medical profession, which does not agree that subluxations are the root of all evil. Contrary to popular opinion, this—and not the flow of patient dollars— is the main bone of contention between medical doctors and chiropractors.)

One major concern in chiropractic has always been to correct improper posture and muscle tightness or spasm, since these can pull the spine out of proper alignment. In the early 1960s, practitioner George Goodheart came to the conclusion that muscle *spasm* was not so much a problem as was muscle *weakness*, which would cause normal muscles on the opposite side of the body to appear (or become) tight. The crucial issue was thus finding the weak muscles and somehow strengthening them. Goodheart appropriated standard muscle-testing techniques from physical therapy texts and combined them with Chinese concepts of energy flow, eventually producing in 1954-71 the *Applied Kinesiology Research Manuals*.

His ideas were popularized by Pasadena chiropractor John Thie as *Touch for Health,* "a new approach to restoring our natural energies." Applied kinesiology has also enjoyed substantial exposure in chiropractic training schools, where it is usually taught on an elective basis or in the setting of an extracurricular club. (It should be stated from the outset that applied kinesiology is unrelated to formal kinesiology, the study of bodily movements and the muscles which control them. The latter is a legitimate science with applications to physical therapy and rehabilitation.)

Touch for Health has become the most popular form in which applied kinesiology has been packaged for widespread consumption, and we will take a look at its assumptions in some detail. This technique can be learned in neighborhood classes or in one's own living room using Thie's manual, which consists mostly of diagrams of muscle tests and treatments. In its opening pages, the book lays some important theoretical groundwork.

First, Thie states his belief that "the innate intelligence that runs the body is connected to universal intelligence that runs the world, so each person is plugged into the universal intelligence through the system."[1] Thus, classical chiropractic therapy, which is said to clear the communication system between the nerves and the body, also aims to improve communication with universal intelligence, according to Thie.

Second, Touch for Health assumes that certain muscles have special relationships with various internal organs. These relationships have no basis in traditional anatomy and can be understood only in terms of meridians and the flow of universal energy (that is, Ch'i). For example, the teres minor muscle, which connects the lower shoulder blade and upper arm, is said to be affected by changes in the thyroid gland; the triceps, which straightens the arm at the elbow, reflects conditions of the pancreas; the anterior deltoid, which helps flex the shoulder, is related to the gall bladder. If the organ is malfunctioning in some way, its associated muscle will be weakened; furthermore, if the muscle can be strengthened, the organ will be on the road to recovery.

How does one decide where the problems lie? One method

Touch for Health recommends is none other than traditional Chinese pulse testing. The manual provides clearly marked pictures and informs us that in feeling pulses, "an expert can recognize a deviation as either too strong or too weak. For beginners, just a difference in the feel will be enough of a clue. With this information, go to the muscles which are associated with the meridians for that pulse, use the muscle tests, and treat the weak muscles by any of the methods."[2]

The more important diagnostic approach in Touch for Health is muscle testing. This is done using standard textbook methods of judging muscle strength, except that, instead of checking for obvious deficiencies in resistance, extremely subtle variations are sought. The first two or three inches of the muscle's range or motion are considered most important, and the examiner looks for either a "locking" of the muscle or a "mushy" giving way as the clue to normalcy or weakness. Testing has another important function, according to Thie: "Unless a muscle has just been used, as in the tests, energies released in treatment have only a general effect throughout the body and do not always give enough benefit to the specific muscle in need of stimulation. Using the muscle first seems to tell the energies where to go and what to do."[3]

The crux of Touch for Health is, indeed, the flow of Ch'i—flowing through meridians, just as the ancients claimed—bringing health when in balance, and disorder when blocked or drained. The new twist is the effect of Ch'i imbalances on specific muscles, which provides a convenient way to diagnose or treat: no confusing attention to yin and yang, no tedious memorization of the five-elements diagram and, best of all, no nasty needles to contend with. Anyone can learn to pull a few muscles, and treatment is even easier. One need simply trace the meridian associated with the unbalanced organ (and its muscle) in order to rebalance Ch'i and strengthen the muscle. The therapist's hand gently moves from one end of the meridian to the other in a continuous motion, and strength is supposed to be restored. Amazingly, one need not even be terribly accurate for this technique to work:

Using the flat of the hand will give better coverage, but it is only necessary to come within 2 inches of the meridians, either off to the side or *even above the skin and over clothing*, for it to be effective. Tracing can be done quickly, but it is sometimes more beneficial when done with more care. Retest the muscle, and if it is not stronger, try tracing in the opposite direction.[4]

It is here that Touch for Health takes a leap into the world of the etheric body, the aura and the magnetic pass. Once we accept the possibility of bringing about significant physical changes simply by waving our hands within two inches of the skin, we bid farewell to conventional science.

If there is any lingering doubt that Touch for Health is grounded in Eastern metaphysics, one need only remember Thie's initial mention in his manual of universal intelligence. That this is not an offhand remark is made clear in an interview in *Science of Mind* magazine in which he elaborates his understanding of energy. When asked, "What exactly are the energies you balance and unblock in your work?" Thie replied:

They are the energies of the universe, taking form in the individual.

To really understand this, we must remember that we are all one with the universe, with the universal energy. When this energy is highly concentrated, we call it "matter," and our bodies *are* that matter. Therefore, our bodies are literally this universal energy, in some of its various forms.[5]

The universe is energy. We are energy. We are one. The articles of faith in Touch for Health are the same as those we have heard before and will continue to hear in the New Medicine.

Thymus Thumps and the Tongue Button

A few years ago we began to hear a startling rumor that reasonably intelligent people were checking for "food intolerances" using the following test. The person being tested extends his or her arm at a ninety-degree angle to the body. An experimenter pushes the arm downward at the wrist, with the subject offering resistance. After this initial test of strength, a certain food is placed in the subject's mouth or simply held in the subject's opposite hand. If the arm offers less resistance, the individual is declared to be allergic to that food, no matter how wholesome it might otherwise be.

As we heard similar stories from various sources, our initial amusement changed to stunned disbelief. The arm-strength test was being used on a surprisingly wide basis as the ultimate indicator of bodily functions. An especially popular demonstration showed the weakening effect of refined sugar when held in a bag in one's hand.

Perhaps the most amazing feature of these discussions of food and muscle strength was the rather relaxed (and sometimes enthusiastic) acceptance of this testing process by normal, intelligent individuals. The issues involved apparently escaped their notice. Few seemed to question the reliability of arm-pulling as a measure of overall energy. (Neurologists point out, for example, that muscle strength is extremely variable in the same individual, depending largely on the person's *will* to resist.)

If indeed a food held in one's hand could overtly affect muscle strength, we would need to rewrite every textbook of physiology. This phenomenon could never be explained according to our current understanding of the human body. We would have to invoke some invisible form of interaction between the food and the muscle. Furthermore, if holding a bag of sugar drains one's energy, what about other kinds of organic or inorganic material? What about the clothes we wear, the chairs we sit on, the tools we use, the bed we sleep in? Could all of these exert some form of invisible influence on our strength?

A noteworthy effort to answer such questions is the book *Behavioral Kinesiology* by John Diamond, M.D., which claims to explain how food, clothes, art, music and the environment in general cause endless fluctuations in life energy, all demonstrable through the arm-strength test. Diamond, a past president of an organization called the International Academy of Preventive Medicine, derived his thinking from Goodheart's applied kinesiology. He insists that the flow of Ch'i (which he calls life energy and which he identifies with the Hindu prana, the Hawaiian mana, and so on) is the crux of all health and illness. His new twist is the idea that the thymus gland "monitors and regulates energy flow in the meridian system" and is thus the crucial organ of health maintenance.[6] (The thymus, located beneath the sternum, or breastbone, is known to play a significant role in immunity, but its regulation of life energy is a theory unique to behavioral kinesiology.)

To determine the strength of your thymus, you need merely place the fingers of your right hand over the upper edge of the sternum and then have someone test the strength of your left arm. Diamond insists that this test is accurate, because, he says, the arm becomes stronger when the test is repeated after chewing a tablet of thymus extract. In general, Diamond is far more concerned with practice than with theory. He comments: "This test-touch process —touching with one hand while an indicator muscle is being tested —is called by kinesiologists 'therapy localization.' How it works is not well understood. Perhaps some energy circuit is completed to the point in the body that was low in energy. We do not know."[7] In a footnote he adds: "It's tempting to offer explanations for the phenomena described in this book. However, I have kept them to a minimum. This work is new, and to formulate theories at this stage would be premature and limiting."[8]

BK (behavioral kinesiology) offers a simple way to strengthen the thymus, should it be found weak. One simply thumps the upper sternum ten or twelve times, and the indicator muscle will become strong. Alternatively, one can activate the thymus by placing the tip of the tongue against the "centering button" on the roof of the mouth. Using these simple techniques during the course of the day charges up the thymus and helps prevent energy drainage from life's assorted stresses. The thymus also appears to be strengthened by positive emotions—love, faith, forgiveness—and by nodding one's head or stretching out one's arms in an accepting gesture, which Diamond dubs the "thymus gesture."

From here we are led through an amazing collection of assertions about factors which influence life energy. One must remember that all these conclusions are based on the arm-strength test, with the deltoid serving as the indicator muscle which provides feedback on the state of one's Ch'i.

Energy is raised by happy faces and lowered by sad faces. It is raised by listening to "therapeutic voices" and weakened by listening to voices of people whose thymuses are weak and energies unbalanced. Energy is weakened by many seemingly innocuous activities in everyday life: wearing sunglasses, having an electronic wristwatch in the wrong position on the wrist, wearing a synthetic hat, hairpiece or article of clothing (only one hundred per cent natural fibers will do), sleeping in synthetic bedclothes, using chemical deodorants and perfumes, drinking ice water, working under fluorescent (but not incandescent) light, cooking with gas, standing in the vicinity of x rays or microwaves, and staring at certain visual symbols. (A Greek cross, in the shape of a +, raises energy, while the Roman cross, or crucifix, lowers it. Life energy also seems to respond positively to the swastika.)

The list of energy-altering stimuli extends into the arts. Muscle testing shows certain paintings and photographs to be energizing, while others have a weakening effect. Classical music generally raises life energy, while hard rock (regardless of volume) lowers it. Even the isolated note C and those in its vicinity drain the thymus, while those farthest from it (such as G and F) energize it.

In the area of food, BK has a field day. One must diligently test food (by holding it in the mouth and checking arm strength) to determine "allergies." As one might suspect, life energy is nearly always raised by "organically grown natural foods," while "non-organically" grown food, or refined and processed edibles, tend to produce weakness. Refined sugar always produces weakness—almost. In case it does not, Diamond has an explanation in terms of *switching*, a term referring to an imbalance of activity between the two halves of the brain:

> Sometimes a person who is switched will test strong with refined sugar and weak with raw, unfiltered, unheated honey. This paradoxical finding is hard to explain. If a person is severely switched (as frequently happens with a teenager who has been listening for hours and hours to rock music), it is almost as if some inner morality in the body has become reversed, in that the body actively welcomes the "bad" and rejects the "good."[9]

This statement raises a troublesome question of experimenter bias. Diamond obviously expects refined sugar (which he characterizes as "bad") to make the indicator muscle weak. Unfortunately, the strength with which a tester pulls on an arm is as much under volitional control as is the patient's effort to resist. The expectations of *either* individual may thus have a profound effect on the results obtained.

In his concluding comments about food in *Behavioral Kinesiology*, Diamond strays into the realm of medical therapy. If foods can adversely affect life energy, we are told, so can medications, prescribed or otherwise. *Everything* in life must be subjected to muscle testing for approval:

> Whenever you are thinking of taking a medication, prescribed or not, just place it in your mouth and see whether the indicator muscle still tests strong. If the muscle tests weak, by no means should you take the medication, for that would be violating the basic dictum of BK—that if a substance tests weak, it should not be administered. You should immediately remove it from your mouth and rinse thoroughly.

> Your body has an innate intelligence. It should be the final arbiter of treatment, not the textbook or even clinical experience. . . . It is my hope and dream that in the future all medication will be tested kinesiologically before administration. Doctors owe this to their patients and we owe it to ourselves.[10]

Here BK is flirting with disaster. We can only hope that no one has tossed out an important medication because of this irresponsible advice.

The Vitamin Test

While *Behavioral Kinesiology* will probably never be a best seller, similar ideas are beginning to reach a large audience through national magazines, whose desire to publish exciting articles may overshadow the need to check the validity of what they print. Take, for example, an article in the 20 February 1979 issue of *Family Circle*, a common member of the supermarket check-out rack. Billed on the cover as "the amazing self-test for the vitamins your body needs," the arm-strength test is presented as "The Muscle Response Test."

The authors, Walter Fischman (a doctor of Chinese medicine) and Mark Grinims (a chiropractor), describe several vitamin and mineral touch points on the surface of the body. The vitamin A point, for example, is the right eyelid; points for vitamins E and C are just under the right and left collarbone, respectively; magnesium's point is the center of the navel. By touching a given point with one hand and having the opposite arm's strength tested, readers can determine their needs for that vitamin. The amount of vitamin to be taken is determined by holding the appropriate vitamin or mineral tablet in the mouth or hand and retesting muscle strength. When enough tablets are held, the muscle will become strong; the dose can be increased until the muscle weakens; subtract one or two tablets from the maximum amount, and you have the correct dose.

How were the vitamin points determined? Why are contact points located on only one side of the body and not the other? How does the body know what vitamin or mineral is being held in the hand? These and other questions are not addressed in the article. The important thing to know is the technique. A fleeting gesture toward explanation is offered in the article's introduction. Under the subheading "The Muscle Response Test—How Does It Work?" we are told the following:

> The Muscle Response Test appears to be related to acupuncture points and the "lines of energy" used for centuries in Chinese medicine to direct the body's own healing powers. It's an example of how the body can be used as a guide to its needs.
>
> Says Dwain Lewis, physical education supervisor, University of California at Riverside: "There are different kinds of knowledge. We have learned to trust intellectual knowledge, but there is intuitive knowledge that is also valid. MRT belongs to the latter kind."[11]

This kind of thinking is ominous indeed. What the reader of *Family Circle* is being told is nothing less than to cast off reason. It is clear that the vitamin self-test is not based on the science of nutrition.

Science has not discovered a magical communication between an undigested vitamin tablet and the body's muscles. No one in the field of nutrition has discovered any vitamin touch points.

Since their defense cannot be intellectual, the authors call it intuitive. This is a catchword in holistic health, and it is used frequently to describe the mode of thinking for the New Age. Rational, linear, scientific, "left-brain" thinking is to give way to the intuitive, creative, subjective, "right-brain" thinking which has been suppressed for so long in the technological age. (The authors seem to have forgotten that vitamins were a discovery of old-fashioned, scientific thinking, not Chinese mysticism.) It is, indeed, an amusing choice of words to call the vitamin self-test *intuitive*. If anything, it contradicts all that one believes intuitively about the human body.

Jin Shin Do

Since acupuncture has attained a certain air of respectability, it has become relatively easy to promote more overtly magical practices by invoking meridians and energy, which are now proclaimed to be well documented by science. One insidious result, as we have seen, is the undermining of critical thinking. In some hands there is a second result: the teaching of overtly religious precepts as a crucial part of Chinese medicine.

We might use any of several books or pamphlets as examples of this phenomenon, but we will illustrate with one particularly emphatic textbook: *Acupuncture, Way of Health: Jin Shin Do* by Iona Teeguarden. Teeguarden and her husband are cofounders of the Acupressure Workshop in Santa Monica, California, and have studied with several teachers of oriental medicine. Jin Shin Do is an adaptation of some basic precepts of acupressure with a strong emphasis on metaphysics. Teeguarden's orientation is clear from the beginning. She states in the preface:

Jin Shin Do . . . aims at a deep release and rejuvenation, through which the higher, or psychic centers can be opened. Jin Shin Do may be studied as a way of understanding basic oriental philosophy and of increasing our own mind-body awareness. . . .

> I hope that [this book] may serve as an introduction to the
> veritable treasure-house that is the ancient oriental Way, and
> help many people to incorporate these magical and powerful ori-
> ental health arts into their own lifestyles.[12]

There is no pretense here of adapting these teachings to make them
compatible with Western biology. Magic and power are central,
and the ancients have provided the techniques. This thrust becomes even more impressive when we note the author's acknowledgment of thanks to "Iajai, my spirit guide," with whom she became acquainted in Japan through the assistance of her husband.

Jin Shin Do is introduced as the "Way of the Compassionate
Spirit." Jin is compassion, the "magic key that unlocks the true
power of our inner spirit." Shin is spirit, the "Tao within us, or
God within us," the "divinely inspired part of man." Do, or Tao,
is the way, as we described earlier, the ultimate reality, the "Door
of all essence." Teeguarden repeatedly stresses that without accepting the underlying metaphysics, the techniques themselves are
of little value: "Important as these [techniques] are, . . . the most
important aspect of Jin Shin Do is a basic understanding, without
which any technique is an empty husk. The understanding of basic
oriental philosophy cannot be separated from the study of oriental
techniques, for, in its origin and development, any oriental health
art is firmly rooted in this basic philosophy or view of life.[13]

The basic concepts of the Tao, Ch'i, and yin and yang are introduced in strongly religious terms:

> The Tao is the primordial, ultimate, and infinite Source. It be-
> comes the One, a unity of forces, in order to manifest itself. . . .
> The Tao remains the One, united, even as, like the lowly amoeba,
> it draws apart into its front and back. Making itself into cosmic
> playmates, the One thus separates into two forces: the yin and
> the yang.[14]

In setting forth the contrasts between yin and yang, she adds:

> The yin-yang principle teaches us that nothing continues for-
> ever, and nothing is inherently good or bad. "Good" and "bad"
> is a dualism having to do with the relationship of events to hu-
> man goals and desires, and is not a quality inherent in the nature

of things. . . .

The goal of the oriental seeker was not to embrace the good and reject the bad, but to embrace all phenomena and non-phemonena, irrespective of their relative merits.[15]

Of particular importance is Teeguarden's teaching on the life energy, Ch'i (she spells it *ki*). Along with the usual pronouncements that the goal of all therapies should be the balanced and harmonious flow of this energy, she includes a most interesting statement:

> In meditation or meditation-in-action (such as T'ai Chi Chu'an or the external exercises of Taoist yoga) one can actually become aware of one's ki. Beyond that, one can feel its flow through the body and even map part or all of its routes. This is how the meridians and channels of acupuncture and acupressure were originally discovered, and even today this spontaneous and intuitive method of discovery is not uncommon.[16]

If this is correct, the meridians were not formulated by hundreds of years of empirical observations but rather experienced as a by-product of Taoist meditation. (Similarly, many yogis and psychics claim to see the whirling chakras described in ancient Hindu medicine.) Under these circumstances, any attempt to understand Chinese medicine in Western, scientific terms is doomed to failure. As presented in this particular book, acupressure is nothing more nor less than a direct expression of Oriental mysticism.

Overtly supernatural abilities may be developed, according to the authors, by using breathing techniques which concentrate Ch'i in the *hara*, or "center of vital energy." Taoist masters who have practiced these meditations are said to be able rapidly to melt a block of ice by sitting on it. Aikido masters are described as capable of driving off attackers simply by using the power of their Ch'i and little physical force. The student of Jin Shin Do, with these examples in mind, is taught how to concentrate Ch'i and then direct it through the hands using "creative visualization."

Finally, we are brought to the core of the book. In addition to the usual twelve meridians, Jin Shin Do claims to manipulate eight additional meridians called the *strange flows*. Otherwise known as the *psychic channels*, these are strongly affected by meditation.

The bulk of the book explains how to use the strange flows to solve various energy-flow problems. Teeguarden then concludes with a reminder of the centrality of mysticism in these practices. We are told that, as we apply these techniques, "we can become more open and free beings, continually growing and unfolding our inner Spirits, and connecting with the Universal Spirit. We do not need to now be or soon become 'perfect,' but we can be basically happy and free, experiencing the Universal Flow—which is love, which is magic."[17]

Guidelines for Evaluation

Our look at the mystical roots of acupuncture, acupressure, applied kinesiology and the rest of Chinese medicine has revealed that, in many situations, patients are being treated on the basis of religious beliefs rather than physiological principles. So the question remains, how can we evaluate a particular therapy? Should someone have acupuncture for chronic back pain, for instance, or is this particular technique occultic?

The issues, unfortunately, are not purely scientific, but have spiritual implications as well. After much study and reflection, we have arrived at some guidelines which we apply to individual cases.

First, we propose that the only by-product of ancient Chinese medicine which has been reasonably validated is the treatment of chronic pain with counterstimulation therapy, using either needles or electrical pulses. If you are considering receiving such treatment, your pain problem should be evaluated by a qualified physician, and the therapist should be someone trained in conventional anatomy and physiology, not in meridians and life energy. This may seem like a trivial distinction when one is merely seeking pain relief, but "energy balancers" may tend to inject their mysticism into the therapy session.

The use of acupuncture for treating other medical problems, such as high blood pressure, hearing loss, obesity and so on, has not been validated (to our knowledge) by any controlled study and is extremely suspect. We emphasize the word *controlled* because of the problems we saw in the claims made for miraculous cures in China. No one was counting the cases which failed, nor was anyone considering what other factors might have contributed to success. Therapists who treat such problems with acupuncture are in the twilight zone of medicine and usually are working from a mystical perspective.

This brings us to our second guideline. We strongly urge that patients avoid any therapists who claim to be manipulating invisible energies (Ch'i, life energy or whatever), whether using needles, touch, hand passes, arm-pulling or any other maneuver.

Objections to Chinese Medicine

Why do we take such a hard-nosed stand? For two reasons. First, we have seen how the invoking of life energy, especially in the spin-offs from applied kinesiology, throws critical thinking to the wind. Therapists who use such techniques have strayed far from the mainstream of objective knowledge about the human body. Their "science" is based on conjecture, subjective impressions, unreliable data and, most importantly, the precepts of Taoism. They stand separate from the scientific community. You will never see muscle testing written up in *Scientific American* or recognized by the National Institutes of Health. We challenge anyone who is involved in this therapy to take a hard look at its origins, its underlying assumptions, and its supporting evidence (or lack thereof).

Our look at Jin Shin Do provided an example of our second objection: the general orientation of the literature which promotes the doctrines of Ch'i and meridians. The overwhelming majority of authors express a distinct spiritual perspective which is some variation on Eastern mysticism or the New Consciousness. We have seen no exceptions to date. John Thie, originator of Touch for Health, proclaims in *Science of Mind* magazine that "we are all one with the universe." Iona Teeguarden tells us how Jin Shin Do can open our psychic centers to experience the universal flow which is love and magic. Hiroshi Motoyama, a Japanese physician, acupuncturist and psychic researcher, is actively seeking to unify ancient Chinese medicine, East Indian kundalini yoga, and virtually all other psychic or mystical experiences into a single "science of consciousness."[18] Psychic healer and medium Rosalyn Lee Bruyere, mentioned previously, claims to "see" auras, chakras and meridians, and manipulates the latter two in her practice. Under the direction of two spirit guides who instruct her regularly, she teaches a blend of psychic healing, spiritism, reincarnation and Eastern mysticism. The pattern is unmistakable. There is no neutral "science" of life energy and meridians, but rather a highly developed mystical system with strong ties to the psychic realm.

What does all this mean? It means that energy therapists, whether they realize it or not, are carrying out a form of religious practice and conditioning their patients to accept its teachings. Indeed, some therapists enter a trancelike state in order to become a channel to direct Ch'i (or whatever they choose to call life energy) into the patient. The idea of the healer's injecting invisible energy into another person may seem innocuous to most (and silly to some), but the results may be anything but trivial. Brooks Alexander, co-director of the Spiritual Counterfeits Project, warns:

> It is not difficult to see that ... psychic manipulation could turn an otherwise benign form of treatment into a spiritual booby trap. The nature of the doctor-patient relationship implicitly involves a kind of trust in and submission to the healer on many levels. For a Christian to accept the passive stance of "patient" before a practitioner who exercises spiritual power (either in his own right or as a channel for other influences) could easily result in spiritual derangement or bondage.[19]

We find it particularly unsettling to see members of the Christian community having their energies balanced by chiropractors and other therapists who claim a Christian commitment and who feel that they are not involved in any questionable practices. These practitioners may claim that Ch'i, yin and yang, and meridians are neutral components of God's creation (similar to electricity and radio waves), available for anyone to use; but they ignore the roots of these ideas.

The products of natural science—the technologies of electronics, biochemistry and so on—can be validated by controlled experiments whose results are not tied to the religious beliefs of the researcher. But the "technology" of life energy is totally defined by the belief system of its promoters: the mystics, the psychics and the leaders of the New Consciousness.

Christian energy balancers present us with a paradox. They claim reliance on Scripture, but they carry out the practices of an occult system. Most are sincere in their desire to help their patients. Unfortunately, they lack discernment, failing to see the implications of the ideas they promote. Some are even dabbling in the psychic realm, diagnosing disease through hand passes or over long distances, claiming that this is a natural by-product of their sensitivity to life energy.

To these therapists we offer a challenge and a warning. Take a long look at the world of Chinese medicine and then decide whether you belong there. Do you feel comfortable as a part of the New Consciousness movement, promoting Taoist philosophy, supporting a system whose basic message is that "all is one," and helping usher in the New Age of miracles and magic? If not, then it is time to stop participating in therapies which lend credence and support to a world view which is antagonistic to the most basic teachings of Scripture.

Part III
Psychic Diagnosis & Healing

The waiting room is crowded, the office is running thirty minutes behind schedule, and the phone lines are jammed with incoming symptoms. Mr. Jones's appointment is drawing to a close with some instructions on managing his recently twisted ankle. As he is leaving the examination room, he turns and utters a fateful phrase: "By the way..." The physician's spirits sink. Mr. Jones continues, "What can I do about these headaches I've been having?"

Mr. Jones is one of many who share the misconception that a doctor can make an instantaneous diagnosis when presented with statements such as: "My back hurts," "I've been dizzy lately" or "Why am I so tired?" The doctor confronted with a "by the way" complaint (or the infamous question at a dinner party: "You're a doctor? Say, I have this pain...") has one of three options, none of which is ideal:

1) Give a snap diagnosis and a (presumably) harmless treatment. The old cliché "Take two aspirin and call me in the morning"

is no comedian's invention.

2) Escort Mr. Jones back into the room and proceed with a detailed investigation of his headaches. This is fine for Mr. Jones but not so fine for everyone else in the waiting room.

3) Ask Mr. Jones to make an appointment to discuss his headaches.

The conscientious physician will usually choose the third approach. This may irritate Mr. Jones, who had enough trouble getting an appointment in the first place and probably has a tight budget. Unfortunately, he does not realize that there are many kinds of headaches, each with specific patterns, mechanisms and treatments. His doctor needs to know how long the headaches have been a problem, what they feel like, how they start, where they go, what relieves them and whether they are worsening. He needs to do a basic examination and may possibly want laboratory and x-ray data. The problem may require a look into Mr. Jones's job situation, his marriage and family history, and treatment may involve medication, physical therapy and ongoing counseling. On the other hand, the cause may be as simple as an outdated pair of glasses.

Mr. Jones's complaint on a busy afternoon would be a breeze for his physician if either all headaches had the same cause and cure, or if the doctor could produce a diagnosis without asking questions, looking, touching or evaluating—that is, if the doctor were a psychic diagnostician.

The psychic approaches a symptom from a radically different vantage point than the physician. The psychic appears to draw on sources of knowledge which are unavailable to (or simply ignored by) the neighborhood doctor. While most physicians have been taught standard procedures for tackling problems, psychics gather information in a variety of ways. Some will ask detailed questions, while others will request little more than a name and location. Some require direct contact with (or at least a look at) the patient, while others prefer to work long distance. Many psychics are given something belonging to the patient, claiming to pick up "vibrational changes" which are left like fingerprints. Some submit drops of blood or urine to analysis by mysterious black boxes covered with at a distance from their patients (absent healing), sweep their hands around them, or lay on hands with varying amounts of force. They may claim to utilize the power of God, the flow of universal energy, the guidance of spirits, or the patient's inner powers of recuperation. They may operate during normal wakefulness, slip into trances or even succumb to apparent spirit possession. They have in common neither age, educational background, nor attitude toward payment for services rendered.

Our society is witnessing a startling revival of interest in psychic events, and the arena of health and disease is a veritable hotbed of activity. Organizations such as the Academy of Parapsychology and Medicine (most of whose members are physicians) and the Association for Research and Enlightenment (founded by the late Edgar Cayce), while not overwhelming in size, actively promote research in psychic healing. Former astronaut Edgar Mitchell, who has spearheaded much psychic research through the Institute of Noetic Sciences in Palo Alto, California, has said that "psychic healers can become valuable adjuncts to hospital staffs, to general practitioners, and to clinics." A survey published in the *American Journal of Psychiatry* in October 1981 indicated that fifty-eight per cent of the medical school faculty members who were polled favor the teaching of psychic phenomena as part of psychiatric training. Books with titles such as *Occult Medicine Can Save Your Life* and *Psi Healing* abound in neighborhood bookstores. The 1980 motion picture *Resurrection* concerned a woman who became a psychic healer following a near-fatal accident; the film's star, Ellen Burstyn, was coached by psychic healer and medium Rosalyn Bruyere.

In part II we showed how Chinese medicine has quietly introduced millions of Westerners to Taoist mysticism. In part III we enter a different ball game.

dials and knobs. They may practice the age-old arts of fortunetelling and astrology, and they may analyze palm creases, handwriting, head bumps and facial lines. They may hold advanced degrees or lack even a third-grade education. Most do not limit their services to diagnosis, but proceed with healing as well. The following is one example of how a patient might become involved with a psychic healer.

The young couple wheel their two-year-old son past the familiar stares in the outpatient clinic of the university medical center. He has come once again to submit to the ominous mass of equipment which will, it is hoped, shrink the hideous protrusion from his neck. Some bleeding from the mouth during infancy had started an endless procession of consultations and surgeries, all leading to the dismal conclusion that a rebellious growth would ultimately prove victorious. The rarity of the boy's tumor is of little comfort to his parents, who struggle to brighten his days between bouts of infection and pain. Despite all efforts, the mass continues to enlarge, outstripping its own blood supply and subjecting its victim to a foul dripping from its decaying edge.

Into this agonizing situation come words of hope from a friend. A psychic surgeon in the Philippines named Tony Agpaoa has reportedly cured many cancer patients by removing tumors with his bare hands. Thousands of Americans have made the long and expensive journey to see him, apparently returning healed and satisfied. A charter tour is leaving in a few days.

The boy's parents have never heard of Agpaoa or psychic surgery, and they wonder whether the boy could tolerate such a long trip. What about the thousands of dollars in air fares and other expenses? On the other hand, nothing else has worked, and their son is dying. It wouldn't matter how strange the treatment or how costly, if only it would help. The father begins to inquire about short-term loans.

As with psychic diagnosis, psychic healing encompasses a wildly diverse gamut of activities, with psychic surgery falling at the more colorful (so to speak) end of the spectrum. Superficially, the common traits appear to be few and far between. Healers may work

7
A Sampling of Psychics

THE REALM OF the psychic healers is an uncharted and, we believe, perilous realm of supernatural forces and discarnate (incorporeal) beings. Our desire is neither to spin sensational tales of spooks and chills nor to debunk all psychic events as foolishness or fancy. We encourage skepticism as a necessity for detecting con games and dubious cures, but we desire even more to create a healthy respect for what Scripture calls spiritual warfare—the invisible but deadly conflict whose battle lines are the psychics' stomping grounds. For this study we need not only the ability to doubt, but also the wisdom to discern.

Olga Worrall: The Grand Dame of Psychic Healing
Far from studio lights and enraptured TV audiences, quiet services in a Methodist church in Baltimore have been the scene of what appear to be some impressive cures. A child's uncontrolled eye movements became normal in three months; surgery for a brain

tumor was called off after studies indicated that it had disappeared; a malignant growth in the throat of a major-league baseball executive disappeared after two visits to the healing services; an enlarged lymph node on the face of a young woman seemingly melted away within minutes of a laying-on of hands. These and other unusual events—including communication with the dead, psychic transportation to other locations (otherwise known as astral projection), clairvoyance, and accurate predictions of future events—are described vividly by America's best-studied, living psychic healer, Olga Worrall.

Like many of her counterparts, Olga and her now-deceased husband Ambrose were both ushered into the psychic realm very early in life. As a young child Olga described dead relatives and made accurate prophecies, causing no little concern among family members steeped in Russian orthodoxy; much of this was offset by her ability to relieve a headache or abdominal pains by a touch of the hands. Ambrose, too, was the object of visitations and the agent of prophecy and healing at an early age. His scientific training, which led to a long career in aeronautical engineering with the Martin Corporation, caused him to analyze the events he experienced and attempt an explanation in books such as *The Gift of Healing* and *Explore Your Psychic World*.[1]

The Worralls carried on a long career in private and, later, public healing (through the New Life Clinic services at Baltimore's Mt. Vernon Place and Mt. Washington Methodist Churches). Olga continues to speak widely for holistic conferences, often presiding over healing services which serve to bring a weekend convention to a dramatic close. While Ambrose was particularly concerned with theory and analysis, Olga participated in numerous experiments to demonstrate her psychic prowess (such as deflecting the paths of ions in a cloud chamber or altering the surface tension of water). She has also been a favorite subject of Kirlian photography experiments, providing researchers with vivid images of rays emanating from her finger tips while in a "healing state."

As a conference speaker, Worrall is quite engaging: bright, witty, rich in experience, down-to-earth (she may refer to herself as "just a housewife" while simultaneously showing slides of dazzling Kirlian photographs of her hands). Her books likewise project a strong sense of optimism and genuine care for those she has treated. She has not accepted payment for her services and insists that any who seek healing cooperate fully with conventional medical therapy. (Indeed, she is one of the speakers on the holistic circuit who rarely downgrades orthodox medicine.)

Unfortunately, these appealing presentations also contain overt themes of spiritism and New Consciousness metaphysics: All is one, a conclusion derived from meditation which yields "pure, passive, nonselective" (but alert) consciousness.[2] Spiritual healing occurs when a therapist becomes enough in tune with both the universal mind and the patient to become a channel of energy from one to the other. The spirit world is teeming with activity, some of which is directed toward those on earth. (The Worralls describe quite matter-of-factly some vivid encounters with spirit beings in their book *Explore Your Psychic World*, a compilation of seminars conducted at Wainright House in New York in 1967 and 1968.) As we have said elsewhere, Worrall frequently expresses her hope that science and religion will "go steady and get married," producing some kind of unified body of knowledge where the boundaries of science and metaphysics merge.

W. Brugh Joy: Guide to the Transformational Process

A radical change in lifestyle led internist W. Brugh Joy from the corridors of Good Samaritan Hospital in Los Angeles to spiritual ecstasy deep in the Great Pyramid of Cheops in the dead of night. As told in his book *Joy's Way*, his conventional medical education (including medical school at the University of Southern California and postgraduate training at Johns Hopkins and the Mayo Clinic) provided ample opportunity for developing disciplined, "left-brained" thinking. Concurrently, paranormal experiences and schooling in mysticism led Joy to experiment with diagnostic hand passes and manipulations of invisible energy fields. (His patients at times were puzzled by unusual gestures during their examinations.) All came to a head one afternoon when a voice demanded in no uncertain terms that it was time for a change.

The voice explained clearly that my vision of being a physician had been distorted by boyhood ideals and by the current concepts of science and medicine, which overemphasized the body and external causes and ignored the journey of the soul. I was to begin the study of alternative healing practices and reach insights Western medicine had not yet dared to dream, insights that would unify exoteric and esoteric traditions and thus form the basis of an integrated approach to the art of healing.[3]

As taught in his book, lectures and seminars at the Sky High Ranch in California's Lucerne Valley, Joy's passion is not so much for healing as for a radical transformation in world view. The most crucial step in this process is the abandonment of fixed ideas about the nature of reality:

The release out of the hypothetical foundations on which all systems of belief rest is the crux of the Transformational Process. We start out entrapped in hypotheses that we believe to be absolute truths. Then, in our transformation, we see that they are only temporary structures capable of teaching only relative truths. . . .

In the totality of Beingness there is no absolute anything—no rights or wrongs, no higher or lower aspects—only the infinite interaction of forces, subtle and gross, that have meaning only in relationship to one another. Absolutes are concoctions of our rational minds.[4]

As one casts off the shackles of the "outer mind," one has the familiar New Consciousness experience of cosmic unity ("all is one"), enlightenment through meditation and contacting one's "inner teacher," and development of psychic abilities, including diagnosis and healing. Joy places great emphasis on the invisible chakra system, training his students to scan with the hands for disturbances in energy flow and then altering the flow through visualization techniques. He postulates that the chakras act as transducers whereby invisible changes of universal energy are translated into physical changes in the body, and vice versa. Overall, Joy discusses specific healings (such as tumor regression or pain relief) only in passing. They are clearly incidental to the broader thrust of winning converts to the transformational process.

Lawrence LeShan: Training Psychic Healers

Unlike many who have joined the ranks of psychic healers as a result of circumstances beyond their control, psychologist Lawrence LeShan entered the field to prove a point. In his landmark book *The Medium, the Mystic, and the Physicist*, LeShan attempts to develop a general theory to explain psychic events such as ESP and clairvoyance. His explanation is revealing. He proposes that a particular world view is the cornerstone of the paranormal in general and psychic healing in particular.

He proposes that our everyday perception of space, time, cause and effect (the "Sensory Reality") is but one way of understanding reality. Equally valid is the "Clairvoyant Reality," a world experienced by mediums and psychics, one whose ground rules are somewhat different. First, in the Clairvoyant Reality "individual identity is essentially illusory."[5] In other words, "all is one." Second, time divided into past, present and future is also an illusion. Events occur in sequence, but they exist in an "eternal now." Psychics in tune with the Clairvoyant Reality thus have access to knowledge of the future. Good and evil are also artificial categories. What happens merely *is*, existing as "part of the eternal, totally harmonious plan of the cosmos" which transcends good and evil.[6] Finally, energy and information can be transmitted between two beings without regard to their relationship in time and space.

LeShan carefully develops the idea that humans are oddly amphibious creatures, living in the Sensory Reality but capable of experiencing the Clairvoyant if they care to (and even perhaps if they don't). He shows some striking similarities in the characteristics of the Clairvoyant Reality as described by psychics, mediums and mystics from all ages. Post-Einsteinian physics is said to lend support as well.

In order to test the fruitfulness of these ideas, LeShan decided to conduct an experiment in psychic healing. First, however, he undertook a careful study of the phenomenon itself. His observations are instructive. Having spent many years working in the field of psychosomatic medicine, he was well aware of the existence of hysterical symptoms and their potential for "miraculous" cures. A personal review of the literature in the field led him to discard about ninety-five per cent of healing claims as the by-product of hysteria, suggestion or fraud. The remaining five per cent, he said, represented a "solid residue" in which "the 'healer' usually went through certain behaviors inside of his head, and the 'healee' showed positive biological changes which were not to be expected at that time in terms of the usual course of his condition."[7]

Pursuing the healers' explanations for these results—which boiled down either to the intervention of God, the activity of spirits, or the transmission of energy—proved to be frustrating as a basis for an experiment. Instead, LeShan studied what the healers themselves experienced and extracted two basic types of healing process.

The first or "Type 1" healing process occurs when the healer "goes into an altered state of consciousness in which he views himself and the healee as one entity."[8] The core of this event may take only a moment of time, but requires the healer to obtain an "intense knowledge" of the Clairvoyant Reality—"such complete knowing that nothing else existed in consciousness."[9] Somehow, this total surrender of the healer to an experience of unity is transmitted to the healee, whose capacity for self-repair then becomes greatly strengthened. "The healer does not 'do' or 'give' something to the healee; instead, he helps him come home to the All, to the One, to the Way of 'unity' with the Universe, and in this 'meeting' the healee becomes more complete and this in itself is healing."[10]

"Type 2" healing, on the other hand, involves placing the hands on either side of the patient's diseased or problem area. A flow of energy is said to pass through the hands and may be experienced by the patient as heat or a tingling sensation. (This hearkens back to the ideas of universal energy. Surprisingly, in spite of the wealth of literature which connects this type of energy flow to the assertion that "all is one," LeShan is reluctant to suggest what Type 2 healing is all about or how it works.)

LeShan felt that the theory underlying Type 1 healing would be the most easily tested. He first experimented with techniques from various mystical traditions for about eighteen months, seeking to teach himself to enter the altered state of consciousness required to experience the Clairvoyant Reality. He then began working with patients and observing the results.

A typical healing encounter was a simple affair, with LeShan conversing briefly with the patient, asking him or her to sit comfortably and to avoid trying to do anything.

> I would then ... conceptualize this particular healee being in both realities at the same time. I would attempt to reach a point of being in which I would *know* that he not only existed as a separate individual inside his skin and limited by it, but that he also—and in an equally "true" and "real" manner—existed to the furthest reaches of the cosmos in space and time. When I *knew* for a moment that *this* was true and that I also coexisted with him in this manner—when, in fact, I had attained the Clairvoyant Reality—the healing work was done.[11]

LeShan's results varied from the negligible to the impressive (such as significant improvement of a woman's arthritis), with a large number of patients reporting that they generally felt better. He also found it easy to enter a Type 2, or energy transmitting, experience, but observed these results to be less permanent.

Having developed his own technique to some degree, LeShan wondered whether he could train others to become healers. Beginning in 1970 he found interested people from various backgrounds who had not had psychic experiences and led them through a rigorous five-day course designed to create the altered state of consciousness associated with Type 1 healing. LeShan gives us few examples, but he was convinced that as individuals and as groups the trainees were able to produce enough positive results to validate his basic conceptual framework.

LeShan's book is refreshing for its clarity and candor in reporting both success and failure, insight and uncertainty. He does not provide direct medical documentation of his healings, but his anecdotes are detailed enough to appear credible. He does not seem naive about the possibility of other explanations for the healings he observed. Overall, his posture is that of the inquirer, and his tone is objective: "This is what I did, and this is what happened."

Bearing this in mind, one must be impressed by LeShan's basic message. He is not merely a healer who happens to believe in Eastern or New Consciousness mysticism. For him, surrendering totally to that world view is what produces the healing. Belief is identical to technique here. Conversely, LeShan leaves you outside the ball park in psychic healing unless you make a total commitment to the world view of the Clairvoyant Reality. There may be no more cogent statement in all of the literature of the New Medicine than his conclusion that your belief system—indeed, the core of your consciousness—must be overhauled in line with Eastern mysticism in order to reap the benefits of alternative healing practices.

Arigo: Eighth Wonder of the (Spirit) World

In August 1963 two highly educated Americans—Henry K. (Andrija) Puharich, a physician with interests in bioengineering, and Henry Belk, a North Carolina businessman—rattled four hundred kilometers south from Rio de Janeiro in a VW microbus to the mountain village of Congohas do Campo. They had heard tales of an uneducated government clerk who possessed miraculous healing powers. The man they finally met, José Pedro de Frietas, was known to all as Arigo—a Portuguese word roughly translated "country bumpkin." He looked the part. Jovial, burly, rustic in appearance but a natural leader, Arigo had been well known in Brazil for years and was beloved to all but certain members of the medical establishment and the Catholic Church.

The American visitors watched Arigo begin his day with a rambling tirade against alcohol and tobacco, followed by prayer, delivered to a crowd of two hundred assembled in his undistinguished, cement-wall clinic. He then entered a small cubicle, emerging moments later a different man. The bumpkin suddenly behaved like a displaced Prussian general, speaking Portuguese with a thick German accent. His eyes at once piercing and withdrawn, Arigo informed the Americans that they were welcome to observe his work closely and that the patients now lining up would be perfectly safe. This bit of reassurance proved to be well timed. The next few minutes are vividly described in John G. Fuller's biography, *Arigo: Surgeon of the Rusty Knife:*

Suddenly and without ceremony, he roughly took the first man in line—an elderly, well-dressed gentleman in an impeccable gray sharkskin suit, firmly grasped his shoulders, and held him against the wall, directly under the sign THINK OF JESUS. Puharich, standing next to the man, was startled by the action, wondered what to expect next. Then, without a word, Arigo picked up a four-inch stainless steel paring knife with a cobolawood handle, and literally plunged it into the man's left eye, under the lid and deep up into the eye socket.

In spite of his years of medical practice and experience, Puharich was shocked and stunned. He was even more so when Arigo began violently scraping the knife between the ocular globe and the inside of the lid, pressing up into the sinus area with uninhibited force. The man was wide awake, fully conscious, and showed no fear whatsoever. He did not move or flinch. A woman in the background screamed. Another fainted. Then Arigo levered the eye so that it extruded from the socket. The patient, still utterly calm, seemed bothered by only one thing: a fly that had landed on his cheek. At the moment his eye was literally tilted out of its socket, he calmly brushed the fly away from his cheek.

As he made these motions, Arigo hardly looked at his subject, and at one point turned away to address an assistant while his hand continued to scrape and plunge without letup. In another moment, he turned away from the patient completely, letting the knife dangle half out of the eye.

Then he turned abruptly to Puharich and asked him to place his finger on the eyelid, so that he could feel the point of the knife under the skin. By this time, Puharich was almost in a state of shock, but he did so, clearly feeling the point of the knife through the skin. Quickly, Puharich asked one of the interpreters to ask the patient what he felt. The patient spoke calmly and without excitement, merely stating that although he was well

aware of the knife, he felt no pain or discomfort.[12]
Thus began a day Puharich and Belk would never forget. Arigo treated some two hundred patients that particular morning, spending scarcely a minute with any one of them. Many received prescriptions scribbled after hardly more than a glance. These contained unlikely concoctions of vitamins, common medications, and outdated or experimental drugs, often having no logical relation to the apparent illness. A few patients received the eye socket treatment, while others watched as tumors or other growths were slashed painlessly from their bodies. What little bleeding occurred stopped quickly on Arigo's command.

There was no trace of sterilization—Arigo usually wiped his instruments on his shirt—but there was never an infection. No one received an anesthetic, but no one felt any pain. The patients never displayed any anxiety, and they simply walked away, even after the most violent surgery. The prescriptions made no sense whatsoever, but they cured leukemia and serious infections where conventional treatments had failed. (They were also strangely selective, working only for the patient receiving them.)

Promptly at 11 a.m. Arigo reverted to his previous, jovial self, remembering nothing of his spectacular performance. After working two hours as a receptionist at a local government bureau, he regained the German accent for another four hours of gouging and scribbling, followed by five more hours that night. The Americans felt as though they had spent sixteen hours in the Twilight Zone, minus Rod Serling.

Arigo's explanation for his behavior was disarmingly simple. The miraculous surgeries and prescriptions were actually the handiwork of Adolpho Fritz, a German physician who had died in 1918. Having completed some postgraduate education in the spirit world, Fritz had reportedly gathered a team of discarnate subspecialists and chosen the unlikely Brazilian as the vehicle for their healing endeavors. Their recruiting process was effective, if not exactly civil. Arigo had been pummeled with a series of splitting headaches and German-speaking hallucinations which were alleviated neither by psychiatry nor exorcism. Only when he yielded and allowed some unconscious healings to take place would the brutal symptoms disappear. The truce was uneasy: Arigo's Catholicism struggled against the rampant spiritism in Brazil, and he dreaded the thought of playing for the wrong team.

Two impressive healings finally tipped the balance. In 1950, while accompanying Senator Lucio Bittencourt on a local political campaign, the glassy-eyed Arigo excised the senator's recently diagnosed lung cancer in the dead of night using a razor blade. (Bittencourt had awakened long enough to see Arigo enter his room, but then passed out.) When Bittencourt's physicians confirmed the results, the senator told the story far and wide, and Arigo became an unwilling national hero.

In the wake of this cure, Arigo performed a startling surgery in his home town. There a woman with uterine cancer had passed the point of no return. A group of friends, including Arigo, stopped by to pay a final visit before her death. Once again the glazed look came over him; without warning he grabbed a large kitchen knife, ordered everyone out of the way, and thrust the blade into her vagina, yanking out a bloody mass after several violent jabs. The woman recovered, and her physician confirmed that the tissue was indeed her tumor. The impossible had taken place in a room full of witnesses. Before long Arigo yielded to the internal harassment from Fritz and the crowds of people lining up at his door begging for treatment.

During a career spanning the next two decades, Arigo treated over a million patents, averaging three hundred per day, without charge. Peasants and political leaders alike (including former Brazilian President Juscelino Kubitschek) came for healing or brought loved ones, and scores of unusual cures were medically documented. He was eventually attacked by Brazil's organized medical associations, although the physicians who observed him in action could only verify his unexplainable successes. Eventually he was brought to trial for practicing without a license, but the only evidence against him was a collection of cures. While he claimed he never uttered a word which contradicted church teaching, his healing power provided so much ammunition for Brazil's spiritists that he drew fire from Catholic officials as well.

Despite such obstacles (including a brief jail sentence), the patients continued to pour through Arigo's clinic until 1971. He had seen a black crucifix hanging in the air several times, and one day he bid a strange farewell to his friends. He was promptly impaled in a violent auto accident just outside his home town.

Extensive physiological tests (and films of his surgeries) conducted in Congohas do Campo by North American researchers under Puharich's direction failed to supply an explanation for Arigo's abilities. Indeed, the flagrant violation of basic notions of cleanliness, anesthesia and anatomy seemed calculated to insure that no explanation would make sense other than that of Fritz's invisible skill. (The famous eye operation was often performed for supposedly diagnostic reasons on patients with totally unrelated problems, like some sort of supernatural grandstand play.)

There can be no doubt that the ranks of Brazil's spiritists—especially the more intellectual group called Kardecists, named for nineteenth-century French mystic Allan Kardec—were bolstered by Arigo's cures. In his book Fuller describes how Arigo removed a liver tumor by hand from a "wealthy lawyer, a solid, pragmatic materialist." The attorney later became a spiritist.[13] Puharich, who has studied other psychics, including Israeli spoon-bender Uri Geller, has no doubt about the supernatural origin of Arigo's power: "I am quite sure there will be other Arigos. It is up to mankind to cease and desist from persecuting these messengers from the higher powers of the universe and to learn the truth from them."[14]

Edgar Cayce: The Sleeping Prophet
Extending through a time and culture far removed from Arigo's, but with some provocative similarities, was the psychic career of Edgar Cayce. For over forty years Cayce diagnosed causes of illness and prescribed therapy with remarkable success in a manner which would be the envy of any overworked physician: he simply fell asleep.

In a typical session, he would recline on the nearest couch and enter a self-induced trance. The name and location of the patient would then be read to him, without any indication of symptoms. After a few minutes he would clear his throat and announce in a firm voice, "Yes, we have the body." Then he would begin the "reading," an explanation of the cause of the illness followed by a detailed prescription which might include a special diet, current or outdated medications, osteopathic manipulations, massage, electricity, castor oil packs, enemas or homeopathic remedies.

Frequently the treatment would seem inappropriate or even totally unrelated to the illness. (His wife, Gertrude, for example, dying of tuberculosis in 1911, recovered on a trance-given regimen of liquid heroin capsules interspersed with apple-brandy fumes inhaled from a charred keg.)[15] Cayce never remembered the content of his readings, which usually included concepts and vocabulary extending far beyond the limits of his grade-school education. He was thus forced to rely on those around him to record what he had said and to implement the recommended treatments. Though often told that his ability would make him rich, he rarely received payment for his services. He was investigated by scientists and reporters alike and, despite skepticism, was never proved to be a fraud.

Early in his career Cayce was plagued by doubts—concerned that his ability, which had been literally thrust upon him, would lead to arrest for practicing medicine without a license; or, worse, that it was a demonic scheme to lure him from the teachings of his beloved Bible. His first fear proved unfounded, and he apparently forgot about his second fear some years before his death. In addition to the diagnostic readings, Cayce's unusual naps produced a massive outpouring of verbiage which affirmed monism, universal consciousness, reincarnation, karma and so on. To this they added some highly original concepts on the origin of man, the lost continent of Atlantis, and the future of the world.

The story of Cayce's transformation from uneducated farm boy to commentator on the cosmos makes most interesting reading, especially in the hands of his literate biographer Thomas Sugrue. Long an associate of Cayce, Sugrue told the healer's story in *There Is a River* (1942) and described his own inner journeys and relationship with Cayce in *Stranger in the Earth* (1948). As told by Sugrue and other biographers, Cayce's early life was marked by several brushes with supernatural beings, most of them unsolicited. In one memorable incident, a woman with gossamer wings saved young Edgar from an imminent beating by his father, who was tutoring him. "If you can sleep a little, we can help you," she said, and Edgar's catnap resulted in his instantly learning an entire spelling book.[16] On numerous occasions he committed school books to memory page by page, simply by sleeping with them under his head. (In spite of this ability, the dream of every schoolboy, he never progressed beyond grade school.)

As a young man Cayce suffered from severe headaches, and while on a business trip in 1900 he was found wandering in a daze in a railroad station. Rescued by a family friend, he regained consciousness in Hopkinsville, minus his voice. Months of frustration and scores of fruitless medical examinations finally brought Cayce to a bleak conclusion: he would never speak again above a whisper. He eventually became a silent assistant for a local photographer (a vocation he would carry on for several years) and brooded over God's reasons for allowing this misfortune.

On two occasions traveling hypnotists were able to cure Cayce's hoarseness, but only while he was in a trance. Some time later a local osteopath, Al C. Layne, went one step further and suggested that the sleeping patient diagnose his own illness. After a few minutes Cayce's voice, strong and clear, explained that the problem was "a partial paralysis of the inferior muscles of the vocal cords, produced by nerve strain."[17] The solution, that of verbally commanding the circulation of the affected area to increase, caused the young man's upper chest and neck to turn flaming red for twenty minutes. Cayce awakened, cured and elated, though remembering nothing.

Thus began an uneasy relationship with Layne, who could hardly wait to try out Cayce's diagnostic skill on himself. The next day Edgar's unconscious voice outlined an involved treatment for Layne's disabling abdominal problems, which improved immensely. The next step was obvious. Layne opened an office of "suggestive therapeutics and osteopathy," reading names and locations of patients to the sleeping Cayce and administering the recommended therapies. Cayce was less than enthused, fearing a disaster. Unfortunately, he was trapped. Sugrue writes, "He wanted to quit, yet he couldn't. About once a month his voice dwindled and faded, and he needed Layne to give the suggestion necessary for its return."[18]

Indeed, Cayce could not carry on a normal existence for very long before the hoarseness or a serious illness among family or friends would necessitate a reading. Eventually the fears and doubts began to fade as he saw the happy outcomes of his unconscious work, often in cases where conventional medicine had proven worthless. The five-year-old daughter of Hopkinsville's former superintendent of schools recovered from near-fatal convulsions; Cayce's wife escaped death from tuberculosis; his six-year-old son, Hugh Lynn, regained his sight after a severe powder burn—all in response to directions given by the readings. Year after year Cayce could not help but be impressed. Yet he remained cautious.

The Bible had always been the authority for his conscious mind, and he was determined to prevent his unconscious ability, which he believed to be a gift from God, from falling under the control of the devil. He had passed beyond the point of questioning the readings themselves. Nothing but good seemed to have come from them, and they were devoid of any metaphysical content which might conflict with Scripture The year 1923, however, brought a startling change.

A wealthy printer from Dayton, Ohio, Arthur Lammers, entered Cayce's photography studio one day with a request for answers to the riddles of the universe. His interests were in the ancient mystery religions, psychic phenomena, astrology, yoga and the etheric world. Lammers barraged Cayce with questions and challenged him to help uncover secrets of life, death and the human soul. Cayce's guard was down. The Sunday-school teacher consented to do metaphysical readings, beginning with Lammers's horoscope.

He awoke from the first reading to find Lammers excited. According to the unconscious voice, Lammers was currently on his third trip to earth. His previous appearance had been as a monk, accounting for his present spiritual interests. Cayce had validated the ancient concept of reincarnation and much more. "The important thing," Lammers emphasized, "is that the basic system which runs through all the mystery religions, whether they come from Tibet or the pyramids of Egypt, is backed by you. It's actually the right system."[19]

After more of the same ideas emerged in a second reading, Cayce was plainly uneasy. He had reached a critical point and wondered whether he should continue. "What you've been telling me today," he told Lammers, "and what the readings have been saying, is foreign to all I've believed and been taught, and all I have taught others, all my life. If ever the Devil was going to play a trick on me, this would be it."[20] After much wavering, he chose to allow Lammers to conduct more readings. The crucial factor in the decision was the accuracy and success of his medical diagnoses. The voice he could never remember had performed with spectacular success for twenty-two years. Who could argue with such a track record?

For weeks dozens of metaphysical readings were carried out, which included some rather improbable interpretations of Scripture, as well as what Cayce began to call "life readings." These included not only an assessment of an individual's personality and talents, but also a detailed account of his or her past appearances on earth and their roles in shaping the present life situation. Some twenty-five hundred life readings were delivered over the next twenty-two years, providing as an incidental bonus an elaborate cosmology, an extensive commentary on ancient civilizations, stories from the Old Testament and the life of Jesus, and prophecies of future events.

Eventually Cayce and his family moved to Virginia Beach, where the lifelong dream of a hospital was finally realized in 1928, only to collapse under financial burdens in 1931. Out of the ruins of the dream, however, was born the Association for Research and Enlightenment (A.R.E.), an organization founded by Cayce and his followers to study the paranormal in general and the readings in particular.

Through the 1930s and early 1940s more and more readings in response to increasing public interest gradually overshadowed Cayce's previously quiet way of life. Although individual readings typically produced only a feeling of mild hunger, by 1944 their sheer number left Cayce burned out. He collapsed, managing only to gather enough strength for a reading on himself. The treatment was simple: go away and rest. Regarding duration of treatment, the answer was blunt: "Until he is well or dead."[21] (Cayce's readings were never strong in bedside manner.) Despite improvement with rest, a stroke followed in one month and death in early 1945.

Cayce left behind 14,249 stenographically recorded readings for 5,772 different people, totaling some fifty thousand single-spaced, typewritten pages.[22] (An estimated 16,000 readings were given during his lifetime, but most of the earliest were not preserved.) These were collected by the A.R.E. along with scores of testimonial letters, comprising what is said to be the largest accumulation of documented clairvoyant diagnosis in existence.

The A.R.E. is alive and well today in Virginia Beach, occupying Cayce's original hospital building, which it repossessed in 1958. From its headquarters and new library (containing over seventeen thousand books on paranormal events) emanates a broad range of activities: methodically indexing, studying and disseminating the readings in circulating files; sponsoring research projects in psychic phenomena; organizing numerous conferences, including an annual meeting on holistic health; and maintaining a clinic in Phoenix, where treatments include some of the Cayce prescriptions. Cayce's legacy thus extends far beyond his numerous trance diagnoses. His readings have influenced the metaphysical outlook of thousands and have encouraged many people to contact the forces which Cayce possessed—or which possessed Cayce.[23]

Spiritual transformation (and not medical treatment) is clearly the focus of the publications which have resulted from Cayce's readings. Gina Ceminara's biography of Cayce, *Many Mansions* (1950), is a manifesto of reincarnation doctrine, and Jess Stearn's *Edgar Cayce: The Sleeping Prophet* (1967) stimulated much public interest. One of Cayce's sons, Hugh Lynn, edited an extensive series of books which presented the readings' commentary on prophecy, dreams, reincarnation, Atlantis, Jesus, and the Old Testament, to name a few. As explained in depth in these volumes, the readings teach a sort of Christianized synthesis of several occult and mystery-religion doctrines (many of which the New Testament epistles specifically refute). They proclaim clearly that "all is one" and that God is universal consciousness, energy, creative forces—impersonal but somehow intelligent. They also repeatedly teach the age-old doctrine of karma: the idea that souls pass through numerous lives on earth (and other "planes") as they evolve toward God, reaping the penalties or benefits accrued in past lives and simultaneously shaping future incarnations. Given enough good deeds in enough incarnations, souls eventually will save themselves as they evolve toward, and ultimately become, God.

Jesus is described as but one of some thirty incarnations of the Master, who also appeared as a variety of Old Testament notables (such as Adam, Enoch, Joseph and Joshua) and as Hermes, the builder of the Great Pyramid of Egypt. Jesus, the man, is distinguished from the Christ, or Christ-consciousness, echoing the ancient Gnostics. According to the readings, Jesus was also an Essene, thoroughly trained in Eastern occult wisdom. The importance given to Jesus Christ in the metaphysical readings was apparently a crucial factor (along with the success of the medical readings) in Cayce's acceptance of their teachings. Sugrue writes:

> [Cayce] had been taught to interpret the Bible literally, and he had for a quarter of a century been teaching a literal interpretation of it to his Sunday School classes. He and Gertrude had finally come to believe in the reliability of his clairvoyance; now that clairvoyance informed him that what he believed about God and salvation was primitive, over-simplified, and in many details untrue; . . . it acted as if the gnostics (an early Christian heresy) had not been defeated by orthodoxy after all; it proclaimed a Christianity so long condemned that to Edgar it sounded like the liturgies of Lucifer, the articles of Confederacy of the damned. Only by its constant reference to Christ as the apex of truth and the realization of every soul did it give him comfort.[24]

For all Cayce's Bible reading and Sunday-School teaching, he somehow failed to acquire (or he simply abandoned) a grip on the basic precepts of Scripture.

While the metaphysical readings aroused widespread interest, the medical readings never made a dent in the scientific community. One reason for this was that, in their raw form, they were nearly incomprehensible. Cayce even had trouble finding a stenographer to transcribe them. The following medical discussion, for example, is taken from a 1932 reading for an eighteen-year-old woman with arthritis:

> In the present—from those glands of the lacteals in assimilation, from the activities from the spleen and those glands from the kidneys, the adrenal and those in the lydin, overactive at times, and those of the pancreas supplying to the bloodstream those forces from the adrenals,—all of this makes for the stoppage, rather than the drainage from extremities. This must eventually cause Sleeping Paralysis or Stony Paralysis.[25]

The passage is no more meaningful physiologically than it is grammatically.

Another reason for lack of interest among physicians was the difficulty of extracting principles from the readings which are consistent with the facts of biology. To explain the causes of an illness, the trance voice usually invoked vague disturbances of internal organs, expressed in terms of forces and activities, assimilation and elimination, circulation and vibratory states. Prescriptions, however, were dictated with cookbook precision and often voluminous detail.

A few physicians have attempted to sort out Cayce's remedies and use them in daily practice. One of the most prominent is Harold J. Reilly, a physiotherapist whose clinic in Rockefeller Center, New York, was frequented by celebrities and politicians before his retirement. Reilly was named hundreds of times in the readings and received over a thousand referrals between 1930 and 1945, eventually developing a close association with Cayce. Upon retirement from his New York practice, Reilly donated his physiotherapy equipment to the A.R.E. in Virginia Beach, then settled on a New

Jersey farm where a limited number of patients (A.R.E. members only) still receive treatments.[26]

Currently, the most active Cayce therapists are William and Gladys McGarey, medical doctors who founded the A.R.E. clinic in Phoenix in 1970. Patients at the clinic are treated with both conventional and alternative therapies, the most popular of which seem to be castor-oil packs. This was so frequently prescribed by the readings, most often for abdominal disorders, that William McGarey was prompted to write *Edgar Cayce and the Palma Christi*, extolling the virtues of castor oil.[27] (*Palma Christi*, or Christ's palm, was the medieval title for the castor-oil plant. Conventional medical literature has contained virtually nothing about castor oil since the 1930s, aside from noting its powers in relieving constipation.)

It should come as no surprise that therapists who use the Cayce prescriptions subscribe, virtually without exception, to the metaphysics of the readings and stress the importance of the patients' doing likewise. Harold J. Reilly, explaining why he eventually limited his practice to A.R.E. members, stated: "If they do not understand the Cayce philosophy of the unity of body, mind, and spirit, and their consciousness is not attuned to the necessary level, it takes too long to get results; sometimes it never happens."[28]

Sugrue, writing while Cayce was still alive, also made a telling point: "Those who have gotten the best results from their readings are those who have realized the spiritual implications of the experiment in which they have participated. These, for the most part, have entered into the philosophical side of the work, and gained mentally and spiritually, as well as physically."[29]

William McGarey, a regular speaker on the holistic health circuit, also stresses metaphysical enlightenment. His lectures and writings contain many references to "universal forces" and "creative energies . . . that some call God." He gleans from the readings a sort of microscopic pantheism, a concept that "each cell has a consciousness of its own."[30] Thus healing is formulated as "an awakening of the consciousness of the cells within the body to the Divine. We try . . . to aim our healing at the person and his consciousness, rather than at the disease."[31] One of Cayce's readings is cited as a proof text. During the application of a wet-cell appliance (designed to alter electrical vibrations within the body), the trance voice recommended that "during the period (of the treatment), let the mind be in an attitude of constructive hopefulness, and know that no medicine, no application—mechanical or otherwise—does the healing, but that only the attunement to the Divine within, brings health."[32]

8
A Check List
for Your
Neighborhood
Healer

IN THE PRECEDING chapter we met a few players on the psychic team, both past and present, who have earned special notoriety. There are many others we could name who have similar visibility and thousands more who have not made speeches or written books but who influence the lives of millions of people. These people confront us with data which contradict our everyday experience. We do not normally expect a touch of the hands to cure serious illness, and we have no way to explain how a Brazilian could jam a pocket knife into eye sockets without causing harm.

The great temptation is to respond emotionally—with thrills and chills, a skeptical smirk, a shudder—and to proceed no further What we need as we approach the neighborhood healer is a fistful of questions. These questions, by the way, are the same we should ask of the newest product from Upjohn Pharmaceuticals or this week's diet in the *National Enquirer*.

What Happens?

How do we know when anyone has actually been healed? The spectrum of possible improvements ranges from feeling a little better to being raised from the dead. We should be impressed when a visible tumor melts before our eyes, and less excited when someone announces that her back is less stiff.

To evaluate results it is helpful to think of diseases in terms of two basic categories: pathological and physiological. A pathological disorder creates definite tissue changes which can be identified and measured. A tumor mass, a cataract, an infected toenail or an inflamed pancreas can be documented with the naked eye, x rays or microscopic examination. Progress or deterioration can be charted accordingly. The physiological (sometimes called functional) problem, on the other hand, occurs when structurally normal tissue misbehaves. The muscles which cause a tension headache would not appear abnormal under the microscope; they simply contract too hard and too long.

The pathological/physiological distinction may have no bearing on the importance of the problem. A wart is a pathological nuisance; a migraine headache is a physiological torment. Unfortunately, physiological problems tend to be very common, very stubborn and very dependent on the patient as the indicator of progress. How intense the symptom is, what emotions it calls forth and how likely the sufferer is to say something about it all cloud the picture. Mr. Brown might ignore his headache during the Super Bowl and gripe about it for hours the next day at the office. We cannot measure his pain, so we must accept his words as our data.

To muddy the waters even more, a patient's expectations (positive or negative) have a tendency to come true, particularly (but not only) in functional disorders. Aunt Sally's chronic fatigue may not evaporate when her internist decides that there is nothing wrong with her, but she may feel terrific after a psychic therapist announces that her life energies are no longer blocked. Her improvement may have a lot less to do with life energies than with the high expectations created by the healer.

Here conventional medicine is over a barrel. Consumer advocates have clamored for the end of the M. Deity posture which says, "Do what I say, take this medicine, don't ask questions, and you'll get well." Now statements of informed consent must spell out the gory details of every possible complication of a procedure; patient information packets warn of side effects lurking in prescription bottles; physicians find themselves uttering a stream of maybe's and might's, forgetting the power of reassurance and persuasion.

The psychic healer or other unorthodox practitioner, by contrast, is often a master at creating positive expectations using warm repartee, elaborate rituals and very specific directions. Ironically, the therapist who calls for patients to "take an active role in their healing" one moment may then present a patient with a treatment plan so bizarre that it can be accepted only on blind faith. "Do what I say, take these extracts and herbs, don't ask questions, and you'll get well," says the New Medicine, borrowing the Old Medicine's discarded script.

The bottom line is this: we cannot assume that a psychic healer is curing disease just because the patients are satisfied. Satisfaction may not correlate with biological change. What kind of illnesses are improving? Are people simply saying that they feel better, or are there objective changes which can be verified by a knowledgeable observer?

What Is a Miracle?
In everyday life we seldom have to decide whether an event is a miracle. For the most part, healers meditate or wave their hands and then claim they have unblocked an energy flow or opened a chakra. The patient usually manifests no obvious change other than reporting a tingly sensation or a general feeling of relaxation. Here the issue is not so much whether a miracle occurred, but whether we accept the healer's explanation for the results, if any. Unless one has bought into the New Consciousness, there may be no particular reason to believe anything the healer says without some compelling evidence.

So what evidence might we consider compelling? One factor to consider is the severity of the problem and the degree of improvement. Interestingly, the one form of healing which would force the issue in a hurry is not a part of the standard psychic repertoire. This is what we might call creative healing: raising the dead, restoring sight to a person without eyes, making a withered limb normal. It is one thing to induce diseased tissue to disappear (or whack it out); it is quite another to create healthy tissue from nothing. George Bernard Shaw once visited the Shrine at Lourdes in the French Pyrenees, where thousands of healings had been reported (some very well documented and a few biologically unexplainable). He noted the stacks of discarded crutches left behind by those who decided they could walk without them and is said to have quipped that a few wooden legs in the pile would have been more convincing. A great many of the healings performed by Jesus were of this creative type.

Even very serious conditions may suddenly change course without the help of physicians, psychics or anyone else. Few examples are better presented than Norman Cousins's *Anatomy of an Illness*, the story of the author's battle with a severe autoimmune disorder (in which the immune system attacked his own tissues). Cousins had failed to improve after several days in the hospital, and with his physician's permission he designed his own cure: a comfortable hotel room, vitamin C and daily doses of Laurel and Hardy.[1]

Every physician has a favorite story of a cancer patient whose tumor disappeared for no apparent reason, or a rheumatoid arthritis victim whose joints calmed down on their own, or a multiple sclerosis sufferer who danced into the office one day after months in a wheelchair. Some 176 documented cases of unexpected cancer cures were recorded in the book *Spontaneous Regression of Cancer* by surgeons Tilden Everson and Warren Cole.[2] These undoubtedly represent only a fraction of the number of actual cases which have occurred. It is worth asking why these cures take place; they represent more than just a lucky break for the patient.

Another factor to consider is the time frame of the healing. If a hopeless situation turns around overnight, we may be out of the bounds of normal biology. But if psychic therapy produces very slow progress, we might ask whether it is adding anything to the body's own powers of recuperation. Too often we forget that the human body is basically a survivor, stubbornly improving even when its owner might prefer that it stop trying. Most illnesses resolve (or at least wax and wane) on their own, in spite of our clever interventions. The knowledgeable physician is not afraid to use "tincture of time" as the primary medicine when appropriate. Indeed, many well-known psychics (such as Lawrence LeShan and Olga Worrall) feel that their treatments simply help the body heal itself, though perhaps they speed up the process.

A third consideration, which we have already mentioned, is the power of belief and expectation. Quite possibly this is the most underutilized tool in Western medicine. Some thoughtful efforts to understand and apply these to clinical medicine have been carried out by cancer therapists O. Carl Simonton and Stephanie Matthews-Simonton in Fort Worth, Texas. In their book *Getting Well Again* the Simontons correctly point out that most people have the unbalanced conception that cancer means certain death.[3] They expect the worst, believing that the body is incapable of combating the enemy within. The Simontons teach cancer patients to supplement standard therapies with visualization (for example, creating a mental image of white cells attacking a weak and disorganized cancer). Their goal is to improve the patients' expectations within reasonable limits, and they invoke no life energies or other mystical forces to explain their results.

The Simontons do, however, encourage patients to locate an "inner guide," a practice we do not recommend. The meditative techniques for procuring the services of a guide, as described by the Simontons and many others, are strikingly similar to the old occult practice of contacting a familiar spirit. Both inner guides and familiar spirits are often said to appear in the form of friendly animals or humans who give advice and counsel upon request. At worst, this may begin to transform patients into spirit mediums. At best, it assumes that one's subconscious is an infallible fountain of wisdom, a naive and shaky presupposition for sorting out life's problems.[4]

When tracking down possible healing miracles, occasionally we encounter two other stumbling blocks: fraud (in which the healer deliberately fools the patient) and hysteria (in which the patient unintentionally fools the healer). There is no more readable discussion of this touchy subject than *Healing: A Doctor in Search of a Miracle* by William A. Nolen, a general surgeon and author of *The Making of a Surgeon* and *Surgeon under the Knife*.[5] Nolen made a determined effort to document a miraculous healing, but his prime subjects—an eccentric healer named Norbu Chen, the late Kathryn Kuhlman, and the psychic surgeons of the Philippines—failed to provide any material which convinced him. He is one of many who have shown that the Filipino psychic surgeons indulge in sleight of hand and phony specimens (usually chicken entrails) in their efforts to convince Westerners of their prowess. (He even submitted to a sham operation on his abdomen.)

Nolen's book contains a superb discussion of functional and hysterical disorders, and he shows how every so-called miraculous healing he saw or heard about could be explained in terms of known bodily function. He concludes that "our minds and bodies are miracle enough."[6] That perspective certainly has merit. One walks away from Nolen's book with a healthy dose of skepticism, wondering if those in search of supernatural healing should pack their bags and go home.

Nevertheless, a few stories remain which seem compelling (or at least troubling), even for the hard-boiled skeptic. Many of the accounts of Edgar Cayce's trance prescriptions and their effects on serious illness are difficult to write off if one assumes the accuracy of his biographers. (Unfortunately, there are few firsthand witnesses alive today.) Olga Worrall and Rosalyn Bruyere have been scrutinized by knowledgeable physicians who have verified some unusual cures.

Arigo stands as an example of a real heavyweight. He was repeatedly observed at close range by trained general surgeons and ophthalmologists, most of whom came away stunned by his abilities. Andrija Puharich and his associates carefully photographed Arigo's eyeball surgeries, and at one point Puharich held the knife handle with Arigo to be certain that no trickery was involved. (Just to make sure he was not overlooking any possibilities, Puharich tried sliding an instrument gently under the eyelids of rats and volunteer humans. He found to no one's surprise that neither rats nor humans could tolerate this for longer than a split second.)

We might ask whether Arigo's American biographers could have stretched the facts a bit. There were, however, respectable citizens (including physicians) from every corner of Brazil and the rest of South America who went on record confirming scores of healings. Even Brazil's president in the late 1950s, Juscelino Kubitschek, issued an immediate pardon when he learned that Arigo was awaiting a jail term for illegally practicing medicine.[7] Kubitschek's action was based on personal contact, not merely on Arigo's reputation. It is difficult to believe that such wildly unlikely tales could be a matter of public record for two decades without a single challenge to the basic facts, unless the facts were essentially correct. Indeed, the questions invariably asked by Arigo's visitors centered not on *whether* he healed, but on *how* he healed. This brings us to our final question.

How Should We Respond?

What should be our posture toward the activities of psychic healers? Should we employ their services in hospitals and ask their assistance on difficult diagnostic problems? Should we relegate them to the status of a parlor-game curiosity or a remnant of our less-enlightened past? Are they showing us a preview of the next level of human evolution? Or are they tampering with forces which are best left alone? Should we embrace them or avoid them?

Quite frankly, the answer depends on our world view, the fundamental assumptions with which we approach life. A world view is usually acquired through a combination of socialization, education, deliberation and the school of hard knocks, and it may be subject to change without notice. We may also proclaim one world view but behave according to another, a condition called hypocrisy (or at least confusion). The categorizing of world views is beyond the scope of this book, but is elegantly presented in *The Universe*

Next Door by James W. Sire.[8] We encourage those who desire to understand some important currents in modern thinking to read it.

One reaction to psychic healers is, of course, that of skepticism. We have seen that in the arena of healing a well-trained eye for the nonmiraculous is a valuable asset. There are those, however, who have adopted a naturalistic world view which as a matter of principle denies (or at least resists with a vengeance) *any* supernatural event, including healing. A thoughtful voice for this perspective is called, quite appropriately, *The Skeptical Inquirer*. This journal is published quarterly by the Committee for the Scientific Investigation of Claims of the Paranormal (CSICP). Originally sponsored by the American Humanist Association, the CSICP denies that it rejects any claims out of hand; nevertheless its contributors (including well-known writers such as Isaac Asimov, Carl Sagan and B. F. Skinner) routinely debunk UFO sightings, biorhythm charts, ESP and astrologic predictions, not to mention psychic healing. *The Skeptical Inquirer*'s scientific reports and witty commentary are certainly worth reading, but one can't help wondering if *any* evidence could convince the editorial team that an event was truly supernatural.

Another interpretation of psychic healing comes, of course, from the healers themselves and their admirers in holistic health. We have yet to come across a psychic healer who does not profess some combination of ancient Eastern traditions, monistic ("all is one") thinking, overt spiritism, or all of the above. Even if the healings are highly suspect (or totally fraudulent), these world views are still conveyed with conviction. (Even with their fakery the Filipino psychic surgeons convincingly promote spiritism through a network of some four hundred centers bearing the title of the Union of Christian Spiritists of the Philippines.)

If the world view of the Old and New Testaments is used as the basis for evaluating the psychics, a totally different picture emerges. Contradicting the hard-boiled skeptic, the Scriptures clearly teach the existence of a supernatural realm with which human beings may interact. But in contrast to the euphoric picture painted by the New Consciousness, the Bible consistently declares the psychic realm in whatever guise to be off-limits for humans.

The reasons for this are numerous, but all arise from the issue of spiritual conflict. Eastern mysticism and the New Consciousness declare that the categories of good and evil are based only on our limited understanding of the universe. There are no absolutes, but only the ebb and flow of the Tao, the cycles of yin and yang, the polarities of the same unity, the light and dark sides of the Force.

The Scriptures, on the other hand, describe a spiritual rebellion against the Creator which eventually contaminated humankind and continues to this day. This warfare is never presented as a symbol of humanity's struggle with itself, but as a direct confrontation between opposing personalities. "I am the LORD, and there is no other; apart from me there is no God," said Yahweh through the prophet Isaiah (45:5). "I will raise my throne above the stars of God; ... I will make myself like the Most High," said Lucifer (Is 14:13-14). Once called "son of the dawn," Lucifer is now known by the Hebrew word for adversary: Satan.

Most of Scripture is concerned with the endless battle for human allegiance to one or the other side of the invisible conflict. The apostle Paul, highly educated in the Old Testament and well aware of the mysticism of his day, wrote to the newborn church in Ephesus: "Our struggle is not against flesh and blood, but against the rulers, against the authorities, against the powers of this dark world and against the spiritual forces of evil in the heavenly realms" (Eph 6:12).

Two strong currents in Scripture have a direct bearing on the world view and practices of psychic healers. One is the consistent Old Testament condemnation of practices designed to gather knowledge from invisible sources and to exercise spiritual power apart from God. The message to the Hebrews, as they prepared to enter the land promised to them, was blunt:

Let no one be found among you who sacrifices his son or daughter in the fire, who practices divination or sorcery, interprets omens, engages in witchcraft, or casts spells, or who is a medium or spiritist or who consults the dead. Anyone who does these things is detestable to the LORD, and because of these detestable

practices the LORD your God will drive out those nations before
you. (Deut 18:10-12)

Isaiah, writing centuries later, expresses similar disapproval with
a tinge of sarcasm: "When men tell you to consult mediums and
spiritists, who whisper and mutter, should not a people inquire of
their God? Why consult the dead on behalf of the living?" (Is 8:19).
Scripture describes such behavior as spiritual prostitution, fruitless consorting with God's invisible adversaries.

The New Testament elaborates on this theme by raising the issue
of spiritual deception. Jesus spoke quite bluntly about the activities
of demons, and all four of his biographers describe confrontations
with them in vivid detail. He predicted that, prior to his return to
earth, "false Christs and false prophets will appear and perform
great signs and miracles to deceive even the elect—if that were possible" (Mt 24:24). The clear implication is that an overtly miraculous event could appear virtuous and be just the opposite.

Other New Testament writers echo this warning. John cautioned
the early church, "Dear friends, do not believe every spirit, but test
the spirits to see whether they are from God, because many false
prophets have gone out into the world" (1 Jn 4:1).

Paul, who not only established numerous congregations but con-
stantly battled against their infiltration by false teachers, characterized his adversaries as "false prophets, deceitful workmen, mas-
querading as apostles of Christ. And no wonder, for Satan himself
masquerades as an angel of light" (2 Cor 11:13-14).

These and other passages describe the invisible enemy of God
and humanity as capable of producing impressive and inspiring
displays which are deliberately misleading. This casts an uneasy
shadow on psychic diagnosis and healing. If one accepts the Old
and New Testaments as authoritative, then one cannot assume that
an insight gained from an unseen intelligence is necessarily true,
nor that a supernatural healing comes from God.

Such a viewpoint does not imply that psychic healers are necessarily deceitful or malicious. Most manifest a sincere care for those
coming for help, and only a handful (primarily among the Filipino
psychic surgeons) appear to be seeking unscrupulous gain. Fur-

thermore, it is certainly unpleasant to think that a physical healing could be an occasion for spiritual subterfuge. But if healing signs and wonders are consistently accompanied by metaphysical messages which contradict the core of biblical teaching—humanity's estrangement from God, God's rescue through the Messiah, and the need for individual repentance and submission to God's authority—then whatever physical benefit results from the healing may be offset by a far more profound spiritual consequence. Jesus never minced words on the relative importance of physical and spiritual well-being: "What good will it be for a man if he gains the whole world, yet forfeits his soul?" (Mt 16:26).

There are, of course, other vantage points from which to evaluate psychic healers, but nearly all represent some combination of the three we have mentioned. A common sentiment we have heard is a sort of modified skepticism: an openness to the possibilities of psychic events, while waiting for some convincing proof or a personal experience.

The problem we face is that it is all but impossible to analyze this phenomenon with total objectivity. The proper uses of a new antibiotic can be found (or argued about) by researchers who are agnostic, Fundamentalist, Hindu or whatever. One's personal world view does not need to be changed for the medicine to work. But one cannot study psychic healers for very long without bringing one's personal belief system into the equation. One will either discount healing claims as unlikely or impossible, accept them as evidence for new dimensions of human potential, or view them as a skirmish in an invisible war.

The authors of this book are no exception. We feel that Jesus of Nazareth, whose credentials included creative healings unduplicated by *any* contemporary healer, was qualified to address the issues of truth and deceit in the spiritual realm. If we take his statements seriously, then we must look beyond good intentions and even good results. The messages which come wrapped around psychic healings, and their deep roots in spiritism, Eastern mysticism, and occultism, represent a far greater hazard than any disease which might be relieved for a season.[9]

Part IV
Health for the Whole Person: A Balanced Approach

9

Examining Controversial Therapies

A number of popular New Age health practices whose spiritual implications are not overtly obvious have stirred up much controversy among Christians. Some see these as helpful (if unconventional) tools which are spiritually neutral; when using them, the worldview of the therapist is the key issue. Others may argue that a New Age endorsement automatically indicates that a practice should be off-limits; scratch the "neutral" surface a little, and underneath you'll find messages which undermine the Christian worldview.

Three such therapies are biofeedback, homeopathy, and iridology, each of which poses a different problem in discernment. We will review these and then offer some basic principles which may be helpful in evaluating other health-related practices.

Biofeedback
Biofeedback involves the use of special electronic equipment to

gain some control of a body function which we normally cannot consciously regulate. In theory, by observing how skin temperature, pulse rate, or even brain waves respond to various mental exercises, one can learn how to improve certain health problems.

In mainline medicine, one of the most widely accepted uses of biofeedback is in the management of headache. Patients with disabling muscle contraction headache (an intense form of the everyday "Excedrin headache") can wear special sensors in order to see when head and neck muscles are inappropriately contracted, and then hopefully learn to relax them. Others who have migraine headache, which is caused by spasm and then painful dilating of blood vessels in the head, may learn to abort a headache by controlling skin temperature. The technique is limited in usefulness by the time, expense and discipline required to master it. In addition, the appropriate mental process maybe difficult to carry out under the pressure of a busy day or a tense confrontation.

Aside from these limitations, one would be hard-pressed to find fault with the use of biofeedback for this type of application. The physiology involved is relatively straightforward, and there is no underlying metaphysical message which must be swallowed for the technique to work. On the other hand, many who use biofeedback, including pioneer researchers Elmer and Alyce Green, have supported New Age thinking. In holistic health, biofeedback has been used as a sort of "electronic yoga," a high tech means for altering consciousness and inducing psychic experiences. British psychology researcher C. Maxwell Cade, for example, wrote in the preface to his book *The Awakened Mind*,

> My work, ...while fully incorporating the basic biofeedback principles and techniques in all their aspects, has branched off into a singular direction and emphasis—that of combining biofeedback training and monitoring with the ancient art of meditation so as to try to achieve a maximal mind-body awareness, this in turn leading to the gradual development of higher levels of consciousness.[1]

Biofeedback researchers who are not enamored with the holistic health movement cringe at such pronouncements. Medical psychologist Larry D. Young, for example, in an essay "Holistic Medicine's Use of Biofeedback," has criticized the holistic movement for oversimplification, exaggerated claims, and misinterpretation of biofeedback experiments.[2]

Even without complaining about biofeedback's New Age enthusiasts, one might argue that functions such as skin temperature and heart rate were not intended to be brought under conscious control, and that attempting to do so is presumptuous. Yet such reasoning sounds suspiciously similar to warnings made many years ago about avoiding flying machines because we were made without wings.

Ultimately, biofeedback seems to fall into the category of a neutral technology, which, like many others, can be used for good or ill depending upon the philosophy of the trainer. It can relieve suffering, prove to be a costly waste of time, or serve as a thinly veiled mechanism to usher the unwary into altered states of consciousness. Anyone who considers using this technique as part of a pain management program should check carefully the credentials and orientation of the therapist.

Homeopathy

While biofeedback has earned some respectability (if not widespread use) among Western physicians, homeopathy was booted out of the scientific mainstream many years ago. Nevertheless, it is widely practiced, both in evangelical Christian and New Age circles, as a form of "drugless" therapy.

Homeopathy dates from 1810, when German physician Samuel Hahnemann published *Organon of Medicine*, an explanation of the principles of a unique treatment system. In essence Hahnemann taught that "like cures like," –that is, a substance which causes a certain symptom in a healthy person will generally lead to improvement in a sick one. In order to minimize side effects (a common problem with many of the noxious medicines used in his day), he diluted active substances to fractions such as one tenth or one hundredth, and later to infinitesimal concentrations. The effect of a material was said to be enhanced by a process of shaking (or "succussion") at each step of dilution.

It should be noted that if a solution is diluted enough times, it will eventually become unlikely that even one molecule of the original material will be present in a given dose. Indeed, the author of two contemporary homeopathy textbooks, George Vithoulkas, has pointed out that as such dilutions the ". . .curative effect (is) not material, but involve(s) some other factor — energy." [3] While not all homeopathic therapists utilize the extreme dilutions, this "life force" concept of homeopathy has found a receptive ear within New Age medicine, which, as we have shown, is fond of manipulating invisible energies.

Yet even though the New Age movement has embraced it, in its earliest form homeopathy and its energy concepts only vaguely resembled the "universal energy" ideas which now pervade holistic health. The latter arise from a mystical worldview which presumes that in our true nature we all comprise one divine essence (and are therefore part of God). Homeopathy, on the other hand, initially was built on a foundation which more closely resembled Original Sin. Indeed, Hahnemann has been described by author Richard Grossinger as a "puritanical Christian" all of his life. [4]

Rather than assuming that our "inner self" is a hidden repository of wisdom and perfection, Hahnemann proposed that at a deep, essentially spiritual level our "vital force" is damaged and distored. We have all inherited a unique "disease core" which is destined to express itself throughout life in a variety of ways. His vision was reminiscent of the Bible's description of humanity as fallen and subject to inevitable decay because of the first man's sin.

While the theological implications of Hahnemann's system may be interesting, the scientific validity of homeopathy is, for all practical purposes, impossible to establish. (Indeed, at its roots homeopathy is fundamentally anti-scientific.) The problem is that classical homepathy flatly rejects the common idea that diseases can be defined, understood and treated on a physical level. Instead, it presumes a priori that symptoms and diseases represent attempts by the body to "vent" disturbances in the deep inner plane without damaging more vital internal organs.

Thus, according to homeopathy, Western medicine's efforts to categorize disease are a colossal waste of time, and its labors in counteracting symptoms (even doing something as simple as taking an aspirin for a headache) actually make the patient worse. Its greatest successes actually create its worst failures. Homeopathy's message to Western medicine is, to put it bluntly, "Everything you know is wrong!" Richard Grossinger, in his book *Planet Medicine*, explains this perspective in some detail:

> If the visible disease is not the disease and if its alleviation is countertherapeutic, then the whole of medicine is involved in a system of superficial pallia-tions leading to more serious disease. Doctors do not cure; they merely displace symptoms to ever less optimum channels of disease expression, each of which they consider to be a separate event because of its location in a new organ or region of the body. The disease meanwhile is driven deeper and deeper into the constitution because its mode of expression is cut off each time. . .

> . . .homeopathy condemns orthodox medical science to a wild goose chase of symptom classification when the dynamics of symptoms in no way reflect the dy-namics of the disease. . .

> ...From a homeopathic point of view, the allopathic medical care provided in civilized countries has driven disease inward to such a degree that we see an exponential increase in the most seriouse pathologi-cal expressions--cancer, heart disease, and mental illness.[5]

The committed homeopathic physician takes a radically differ-ent approach to disease. He or she pays scrupulous attention to all of the patient's symptoms, even the most trivial ones. Then an effort is made, utilizing personal experience and the extensive Homeopathic Repertory, to find a specific remedy which produces symptoms most exactly like that of the patient.

When given in extremely dilute doses, the remedy theoretically works in the arena of the "vital force" to help the body dispel its pattern of disturbances. The patient's sense of feeling better or worse afterwards is not nearly as important as the next collection of symptoms. These must be assessed again in order to find the remedy which will help the body work through the next phase of the disturbance. There is no cure, but only an ongoing succession of symptom patterns and specific remedies.

This endless process vaguely resembles classical Freudian psychoanalysis, in which it was assumed that years of work with a therapist would be necessary for anyone to deal with the mental glitches we all seem to develop early in life. Whether the person being analyzed felt any better after a given session was irrelevant, as long as he or she stuck around for the entire course of therapy.

Nowadays the old-school psychoanalysts treat only a small fraction of those who seek psychological help, partly because we are geared today to expect short term therapy, quick fixes and "one-minute managing." Similarly, since we tend to want and expect "fast-fast-fast relief" from our ailments, it is likely that few homeopaths treat their patient in the tedious, long-term process described above.

Nevertheless, homeopathy's heritage virtually eliminates the possiblity of scientific study. Normally a therapy is evaluated by comparing a group of patients which is treated with a similar group which is not. The conclusions obtained are routinely scrutinized, often challenged, and sometimes revised in the open forum of scientific journals and conferences. But how can you compare "treatment" and "non-treatment" groups when disease categories are meaningless and when no two patients can be treated in the same way? How can the effects of a treatment even be measured when you cannot reliably use the patient's physical status as a guide to your progress?

Indeed, in this respect homeopathy brings to mind the logic of conspiracy theories of history. In a conspiracy theory, all world events are said to be engineered by powerful, ultra-secret group (e.g., the "Illuminati"). Any major event which appears inconsistent with the goals of the conspiracy can still be explained in a way which fits the theory. Likewise, in homeopathy Hahnemann's precepts form a self-enclosed core of material which is resistant to revision based on contrary evidence. If the patient improves, the treatment worked. If he or she worsens, the treatment is merely affecting the way in which the inner disturbance is "ventilating" itself. Any result can be explained by the theory. (In some cases, this assumption could be disastrous. If signs of critical illness are misinterpreted as another "ventilation," a patient could be ushered into a premature grave.)

Christian and non-Christian alike may be drawn to homeopathy because of its emphasis on the body's efforts to heal itself and its shunning of drugs and surgery. A few enthusiastic Christians argue that Hahnemann's system is a gift from God, an answer to the medical establishment which they view as steeped in secular humanism. Others, ourselves included, are uneasy with homeopathy's comfortable adoption by New Age medicine and its de facto support of universal energy ideas. Indeed, in contemporary homeopathy the New Age concept of the mystical life energy is often invoked as the explanation for this practice.

Overall, those on each side of the argument should invoke "guilt by association" with some discretion. The fact that humanistic and evolutionary theories can be found in most medical schools does not invalidate the bulk of the information taught (anatomy, physiology, etc.) or the method by which it was obtained. Likewise, the fact that the New Age movement has seized upon an idea such as homeopathy is not necessarily cause for immediate rejection, but it should be an indication to proceed with extreme caution.

Ultimately, homeopathy's greatest weakness is one shared by several other systems: it stands or falls on a concept which is at odds with the mainstream of knowledge about human physiology, and which is resistant to independent validation. Since it is reasonable to assume that God's creation operates on consistent principles which are open for all to understand and apply, we would offer the following principle for discernment to those who are attracted to homeopathy: "Beware of those who proclaim, 'Everyone is wrong except us.' "

Iridology

If one were looking for a New Age practice which could easily be proven to be either factual or fraudulent, iridology would, at first glance, look like the right choice. Instead of mystical energies or invisible channels, iridology studies the human iris, the colored portion of the eye which controls the amount of light arriving at the retina. According to iridologists, the iris also displays in some detail the status of every organ system in the body. By comparing photographs of the patient's iris with elaborate diagrams, the practitioner not only can detect malfunctioning body parts, but also can predict where trouble is brewing before it appears.

Like homeopathy, iridology was born in Europe. A Hungarian physician, Ignatz von Peczely, in 1881 first published charts of the iris based upon many clinical observations. (These were inspired by a childhood episode in which he accidently broke the leg of a pet owl and subsequently noted a distinct change in the bird's iris.[6]) The practice eventually spread through Europe and then to North America. According to *The Holistic Health Handbook,* there are approximately 10,000 iridologists in Europe and 1,000 in the U.S.[7] In recent years the most widely-quoted American iridologist has been Escondido chiropractor Dr. Bernard Jensen, who has written two voluminous textbooks on this subject.

If the iris is indeed blessed with such enormous diagnostic potential, why is iridology not taken seriously in the scientific community? Certainly it should be a relatively simple matter to photograph the irises of patients with known diseases, and map the results. If accurate, this approach could save billions of dollars in unnecessary tests every year.

In fact, iridology is taught neither in medical schools nor in high school biology classes, nor is it practiced (with very rare exception) by optometrists or ophthalmologists. As with many alternative therapies, there are two fundamental reasons for this wholesale lack of acceptance: iridology's basic premise is highly suspect, and its performance has not earned a passing grade using ordinary methods of scientific investigation. The issue is not economics, politics or closed minds, but rather the question of knowledge: on this planet, how do we go about demonstrating that a biological theory is valid?

As long as we assume that the natural realm follows basic principles and is not totally unpredictable, then any of us should be able to learn what those principles are. We should be able to propose a theory, design a way to test it, and adjust or discard our theory if supporting evidence is lacking. Problems will arise, however, if we can't agree on methods for collecting and interpreting evidence, or when we trash evidence because it doesn't support a theory we like.

With iridology there are both theory problems and evidence problems. One major theory problem is the assumption that the iris' connections with the central nervous system allow detailed messages to be sent to it from the rest of the body. (A variation on this idea occurs in reflexology, in which stimulation of different areas of the foot or hand is said to affect distant organs such as the kidney or lung.) Unfortunately, the elaborate neurologic pathways necessary for such a powerful capability have yet to be demonstrated, or even deemed plausible, in spite of years of neuroanatomical studies of the eye and central nervous system.

Iridologists have generally sidestepped the neurological details of their practice in favor of a simpler observation that the iris is indeed connected with the autonomic nervous system. But merely being connected to the system does not prove that all of the body can be monitored. My telephone is connected to a massive communications network, but it does not send me messages about the equipment or conversations of everyone in America.

The notion that one small part of the body can reveal or control all of the rest certainly is appealing—but the appeal is to a universal human appetite for short cuts to knowledge and power. It would indeed be nice if we could diagnose illness simply by looking at the iris instead of laboring through a history, physical examination and a battery of tests. It would be wonderful if we could actually heal a patient's liver or stomach by massaging the feet. It would be life-changing if we could truly understand our future by having our palms read, our horoscopes cast, or our tea leaves examined.

We all want to understand and influence cause and effect. We especially want to know, if all is not well, why we are not up to par and what will make us better. Unfortunately, those answers are not often simple, even when they are available. Establishing how things work in our world and in our bodies is usually a difficult, tedious process, though not an impossible one. Iridology's failure to be taken seriously in the scientific community arises largely because its practitioners have tried to bypass this process.

Another fundamental theory problem for iridology is its insistence that each iris reveals what is happening on its particular side of the body. (That is, the right iris shows right-sided problems, and similarly for the left.) This contradicts a fundamental observation that incoming nerve impulses from one side of the body nearly always cross to the opposite side on their way to the brain. Dr. Jensen has proposed, in response to this problem, that the optic nerve serves as the final messenger between the nervous system and the iris. This explanation would allow for a second crossing of information back to the eye on the same side of the body, but creates two new problems. First, the optic nerve has been shown without question to be only a "one way" messenger, carrying information from the retina to the brain and not in reverse. (Indeed, the optic nerve is not known to connect directly to the iris at all.) Second, only half of the fibers of the optic nerve cross to the opposite side of the brain.

Since the precise way in which the iris tells us about distant organs is at best poorly defined, iridology characterizes itself as an "empiric" science. That is, it is based upon the experience of its practitioners rather than controlled studies. Presumably, over the years iridologists have noted the appearance of the irises in many patients and then correlated these observations with the patients' health problems. Unfortunately, however, iridologists use disease classifications which are not generally accepted outside of the subculture in which they practice. Terms such as "toxic accumulations" or "lymphatic congestion" abound in iridology literature, but they are at best vaguely defined and at worst meaningless to the health care community at large.

This problem is vividly illustrated by the controversy surrounding the only controlled study of iridology in the American medical literature. Researchers at the University of California, San Diego allowed three iridologists (including Dr. Jensen himself) and three ophthalmologists to study iris photographs of 143 subjects, of whom 48 had overt kidney failure. When the number of false positives (normal people who were picked as having disease) and false negatives (diseased people who were picked as being normal) were compared to the number of correct answers, the level of accuracy was found to be worse than chance.[8] In other words, all six doctors would have been more successful picking their answers out of a hat than deriving them from the iris photographs.

Dr. Jensen later criticized this study, arguing that its use of the serum creatinine level to demonstrate kidney disease was invalid. Yet serum creatinine is used and accepted worldwide as a meaningful indicator of kidney function. Furthermore, iridologists have a ready-made explanation for overdiagnosing disease which certainly occurred in the San Diego study in that they claim the ability to discern "subclinical" disease which will cause trouble in the future. But once you claim to be a health prophet, all bets are off. If the patient never develops the problems, you claim that your treatment prevented it. If he or she does, you were right all along.

In short, iridology has the same trappings of a closed system that we saw in homeopathy. Like some sort of "alternate reality," it operates with a vocabulary and internal logic which effectively shut out any challenge from the outside. In addition, its most visible proponent, Bernard Jensen, has given clear notice of his positive orientation to the New Age movement. His most recent textbook (Iridology: Science and Practice in the Healing Arts, Vol. II), for example, ends with an invitation entitled "A Deeper Look," in which he provides an extensive bibliography that is heavily laden with New Age material. His list of "books which have helped me" includes foundational New Age works such as Isis Unveiled by medium H.P. Blavatsky, The Aquarian Conspiracy by Marilyn Ferguson, The Roots of Conciousness by parapsychologist Jeffrey

Mishlove, and the spiritistically received book *A Course in Miracles*. In addition, he lists numerous titles which expound on "universal energy" themes, such as *Human Energy Systems* by psychic Jack Schwarz, *Breakthrough to Creativity* (a study of psychic abilities) by Shafica Karagulla and *Radionics and the Subtle Anatomy of Man* by David V. Tansley.[9]

Nevertheless, one might ask, "So what?" If people are helped, what does it matter whether or not iridology or homeopathy can be validated by conventional scientific methods? And so what if some therapies are popular with New Agers? Isn't the true bottom line the roster of satisfied clients who swear that these systems succeeded where orthodox medicine failed? We asked the same question of psychic healing: doesn't the end result override any other concerns?

The problem with psychic healing, we noted, is the spiritual baggage which ultimately makes the cure more hazardous than the disease. The problem with iridology, homeopathy and other self-contained systems is not that people might feel better, but that their understanding of why they feel better can become grossly distorted. Worse, such a process can open them in a powerful way to the spiritual no-man's-land of New Age thinking. For many this is a round-about route to the psychic realm and its attendant hazards (ranging from theological derailment to outright occult bondage). The first steps on this slippery path can be taken in a number of ways.

First, New Age practitioners will often make the right recommendations for the wrong reasons. An arm-pulling "allergy test" may lead to a diet free of sugar. A homeopath may recommend favoring fruits and vegetables instead of burgers and steaks. An iridologist may see an ominous spot on the iris which sends a patient's cigarettes to the trash can. Most people will feel better with such advice, whether or not the rationale makes any sense.

Second, many patients who consult holistic healers have symptoms (such as chronic fatigue) for which the busy family doctor may have neither immediate cure nor great interest. On the other hand, New Age practitioners more often have the time and empathy to hear the patient out, which is therapeutic in itself. They also invariably find a "cause" or the symptoms, which is reassuring ("Thank goodness, I'm not crazy after all..."). And, most importantly, they usually have a specific and detailed treatment plan, which creates a most important ingredient: expectation of improvement. When we feel poorly, we don't want to hear feedback such as "I can't find anything the matter with you go lose some weight." But our spirits quicken when we hear, "I've found what's wrong, and I have the answer!" The fact that someone finally appears to understand, and can offer help, taps into powerful emotions which tend to override any intellectual or spiritual cautions about the details of the treatment.

Third, and most importantly, in health and disease most of us have a tendency to believe in the concept which lawyers call "proximate cause." That is, if we become sick we look for something to blame within the last day or so. Likewise, when we feel better we give credit to the most recent remedy we tried or the last doctor we visited. If we feel better after seeing a holistic healer, we will probably accept his or her explanation, however far-fetched it might be. This may lead to return visits in the future, and perhaps a growing interest in other facets of New Age medicine.

So many themes and variations come and go in holistic health that a detailed critique of each is impossible in a book of this size. Indeed, we would encourage other interested evangelical writers to review areas of New Age medicine which we could only mention in passing. The tendency for such practices to be accepted uncritically by Christians (or anyone else) cannot be reversed if opposing viewpoints are unavailable.

In an effort to fill some of the remaining gap, we would like to conclude this chapter by offering a number of general principles. These may help guide those who are considering whether or not to become involved in a particular therapy. In honor of the ancient Latin phrase "caveat emptor" that is, "let the buyer beware" we have listed them as caveats. Please note that many of these apply to unusual therapies which may have nothing to do with the New Age movement, but which merely are part of the long and glorious tradition of quackery.

Caveat No. 1: Beware of therapies which claim to manipulate "invisible energy."

We have explored the realm of invisible energies specifically in Chapter 3, and in other places throughout this book. At best, these ideas lack meaningful scientific support, although they may be expressed using all sorts of technical jargon and even equipment. More often, they are based upon, illustrate or validate the core teachings of the New Age: "All is One" and "We are all God." At worst, the energies involved may be demonic in origin, and thus pose a threat rather than a benefit to health.

Christians therapists may claim that the invisible energies they purport to influence are part of God's creation, but in doing so they betray a misinformed notion of the scope of the natural realm. They are, in fact, toying either with the supernatural or an illusion.

Caveat No. 2: Beware of those who seem to utilize psychic knowledge or power.

We have reviewed the hazards of involvement in psychic diagnosis and healing in the preceding two chapters. Nevertheless, as with universal energies, some Christians are tempted to explore psychic capabilities which they feel are neutral ground. Remember that the psychic realm is neutral ground for humans in the same way that a swamp full of alligators is neutral ground for a water-skier. Scripture has posted a clear "No Trespassing" sign here (Deut. 18:9-12).

Caveat No. 3: Beware of a practitioner who has a therapy with which no one else is familiar.

Scientific inquiry is not based on secrets and exclusive therapies, but on the free flow of information and review by independent peers.

Someone with a "secret formula" usually keeps it a secret for two reasons: he or she has some of it to sell you (with a fat price tag), and independent analysis would show it to be worthless. This Caveat has two important corollaries:

A. Beware of those who promote their "discovery"

to the general public (usually via best-selling books) before it is validated by the mainstream of science. If they can't wait to get it out to John and Jane Q. Public, there is probably a good reason: it won't hold water when experts review it.

B. Head for the exit immediately when someone claims that the medical establishment is evil or satanic, that the government and the A.M.A. are persecuting them, or that other doctors are intent on stealing their discovery. Such an individual is due for an appointment with the state Board of Medical Quality Assurance, a competent psychiatrist, or perhaps Rod Serling. Stick around only if you are seeking a visit to the Twilight Zone.

Caveat No. 4: Beware of someone who claims that their particular therapy will cure anything.

You can only solve so many construction problems with a hammer. An important skill of caring practitioners is knowing when, and to whom, to refer a patient with a disorder which is beyond their expertise.

This problem plagued chiropractic practitioners for many years, and still remains to be settled for some to this day. Early chiropractic theory held that virtually every health problem (including heart failure, kidney disease, diabetes, etc.) was caused by misalignments of the spine, and that adjustments would thus benefit anyone and everyone. Such claims are completely unsupportable, and fortunately the majority of chiropractors restrict their attention to musculo-skeletal problems.

There remain, however, a number of practitioners who have reworked some of the old "vital nerve energy" ideas into a broader scope under New Age influence. We know of chiropractors who have blended their practice with numerous other methodologies, including energy channeling, meditation, aura work, Christian Science, psychic healing and overt spiritism. We would exhort committed evangelical chiropractors not only to shun such practices but actively oppose them in their own professional community.

Caveat No. 5: Beware of someone whose explanations don't make sense.

If a physician, or any therapist, speaks in "doctorese" instead of English, stop and ask for a translation. Even the most complex problem can be explained in terms that anyone can comprehend. But if the explanation sounds far-fetched, seek some additional input elsewhere. A term like "neuromusculostructural tensegrity" sounds impressive—but it in fact refers to a localized, southern California synthesis of applied kinesiology, kundalini yoga, acupressure, chiropractic, and something called "mentastics," among other things.

Years ago one of us (PCR) received a call from a man who was questioning a particular doctor's practice. The doctor claimed to be able to diagnose tuberculosis, tumors, pregnancy and nutritional deficiencies from a polaroid picture of the patient. Amazingly, as the patient was treated (with something called "Nana Rays"), the picture would automatically show the results. He asked me what I thought of this, and I asked if any of it made sense to him. He said it didn't, and he was right. The caller could have kept quite a bit of money away from Dr. Polaroid (who has since been sent packing by state authorities) if he had paid attention to his own common sense.

Caveat No. 6: Beware of therapies whose primary proof consists of the testimonies from satisfied customers.

While there is certainly some validity to success stories and word of mouth advertising, the ultimate proof of nearly every pudding is the outcome of controlled studies. Why? Because people can feel better (or worse) for many reasons which have nothing to do with the treatment they were given. Well-designed studies simply try to isolate the effect of the treatment from everything else which may affect the outcome.

We do not, by the way, wish to convey a cultish commitment to naturalistic science in the face of healing interventions by God. God's overriding of the normal processes of his creation are not controllable or reproducible. On the other hand, careful scientific inquiry can help us determine whether a true miracle has indeed occurred.

Caveat No. 7: Beware of therapies which rely heavily on altered states of consciousness.

The New Age movement promotes the notion that ordinary waking consciousness limits our potential. As we have seen, many holistic therapies are built on the idea that healings will occur, or important insights gathered, when we shut down the rational mind for a while (through meditation, chanting, yoga, hypnosis, sensory deprivation tanks, etc.) and experience an "alternate reality." Such experiences are, in fact, critical if one is to accept a number of New Age concepts (especially "All is One") which otherwise lack much support from everyday living. They are also a "no-man's land" in which one may encounter spirit "guides" or become convinced of one's own deity.

Scripture puts no premium whatsoever on altered states, but assumes that we will interact with our creator using an alert, conscious mind.

Caveat No. 8: Sincerity is no guarantee of legitimacy.

The most warm-hearted, sincere therapist may be sincerely wrong. Worse, a cozy bedside manner may delay the patient's recognition that a practitioner has other agendas or a personal commitment to New Age/occultic practices.

This caveat has two important corollaries:

A. A therapist's expression of evangelical commitment is no guarantee of legitimacy either. This is indeed lamentable, but true. Highly visible, church-going scripture-quoting (and, yes, sincere) practitioners can and do lead many in the church straight into New Age thinking.

B. The endorsement of a therapist (or therapy) by a renowned evangelical pastor, speaker, author or celebrity is, alas, also no guarantee of legitimacy. These individuals should know better, but they often do not apply the same rules of discernment to a health situation that they would to a "spiritual" one.

152

In summary, if and when an unorthodox therapy is offered as a solution to your health problem, do not hesitate to investigate fully and critically its roots, history, contemporary forms and promoters before submitting to it or recommending it to others.

Caveat No. 9: "Caveat venditor": in other words, "Let the seller beware."

We have directed all of our previous warnings to the consumers of health care. Our final comments are directed toward practitioners. Anyone who cares for the health needs of others has an enormous responsibility to maintain basic standards of quality. Those who offer practices to the public which are scientifically unsound (or bankrupt) and potentially dangerous are ultimately accountable to their patients. Where personal integrity falls short, the legal system, for better or worse, is forcing the issue of accountability in ways which were undreamed of twenty years ago. How aggressively it will deal with unfavorable outcomes in holistic health remains to be seen.

For the New Ager who sincerely and enthusiastically believes in the spiritual messages of holistic health, we offer a loving challenge to consider the life and claims of Jesus Christ at face value. We are not gods, or part of God, but men and women who are estranged from our Creator. Jesus Christ has made that reconciliation possible through his death on the cross. Only after we surrender our quest for godhood to him can true enlightenment and fulfillment be experienced.

For the evangelical Christian who promotes New Age practices without paying attention to their spiritual implications, we offer an exhortation: you should know better. If the scriptures are new to you, ask a seasoned believer or pastor to help you apply their teachings to your therapies. If you are indeed familiar with the scope of biblical teaching, you have greater accountability to God for endangering the spiritual health of others. The apostle Paul warned, "See to it that no one takes you captive through hollow and deceptive philosophy, which depends on human tradition and the basic principles of this world, rather than on Christ" (Col. 2:8). Be careful that you are not the one who is taking the captives.

10
Alternatives
to the
New Medicine

WE BEGAN OUR TOUR of the holistic health movement by noting that some serious criticisms have been leveled recently at Western medicine and its delivery system. Many of these rebukes are well deserved. Some are misdirected. Most of them have helped fuel the growing interest in alternative health practices. It is our conviction that neither Western medicine nor the holistic health movement can rightly claim to have cornered the market on solutions to suffering or keys to health.

Western medicine is now facing some difficult challenges because of its preoccupation with its greatest strength—crisis intervention. The system's prowess in finding pathology, treating acute illness, repairing injury and sustaining life is rarely challenged, even by holistic enthusiasts. In *Occult Medicine Can Save Your Life*, C. Norman Shealy warns readers that they should "FIRST SEEK COMPETENT MEDICAL CARE for any ailment. Then FOLLOW YOUR MEDICAL ADVICE—it's worth your life. Other help (such as prayer, faith healing, the occult) is very valuable—but only when there is no risk."[1] Shealy seems to be saying that occult medicine can save your life—as long as you're not really sick.

There is no question that we both need and should be grateful for the sophisticated, acute-care system which Western research and technology have created. But some have argued convincingly that acute-care medicine is not actually responsible for improved health in the population at large. As early as 1959, microbiologist René Dubos proposed in *Mirage of Health* that the antibiotics he helped develop played much less a role in gaining control of infectious diseases than did social, nutritional and public health advances.[2]

More recently, Thomas McKeown studied three hundred years of public health statistics in England and concluded that factors unrelated to medicine—such as increased food supply, sanitation and decreases in population growth rates—were the primary cause of improved health nationwide.[3] Furthermore, in developed countries the leading causes of illness and death have shifted from acute problems (such as infection) to chronic, lifestyle-related disorders: cardiovascular and cerebrovascular disease (damage to the heart and brain from impaired circulation), cancer, alcohol and drug abuse, hypertension (that is, high blood pressure) and so on.

Fire Fighting vs. Fire Prevention

An analogy might be helpful here. Everyone recognizes the need for fire fighters and continued improvements in fire-fighting technology. But these are of limited value if most adults smoke in bed, if children are encouraged to experiment with matches and if building codes are nonexistent. In fact, most of us hear so much about fire prevention that it is a rare event actually to see a major blaze.

Our system of medical education still trains new physicians primarily to be fire fighters. Medical students, interns and residents are geared from day one to derive great satisfaction from discovering pathology (or taking a look at that which someone else has found). A complex problem presented on teaching rounds may be called a "great case," even though the patient is suffering terribly. Any interest which the doctor in training might have in exploring the patient's attitudes and emotions will usually be buried under an uncivilized schedule and lack of sleep.

Most physicians are not, in fact, unfeeling technicians with a search-and-destroy mentality which dehumanizes patients. However, the vast majority do find fire fighting more interesting, challenging and rewarding than trying to influence their patients' long-term behavior. Most patients unknowingly reinforce this preference by expressing requests (subtle or otherwise) that something be done to them or for them—and the sooner the better. A minor but common example is the busy executive who wants "something to knock out this cold I've got" and becomes frustrated when the doctor appropriately offers the same advice the patient's mother could have given for the cost of a telephone call.

A more troublesome situation is the young adult who complains of fatigue, headaches and episodes of dizziness over a period of several months. Evaluating such symptoms can frustrate patient and physician alike, because all too often a small fortune is spent on time-consuming exams, x rays and laboratory tests which reveal no abnormalities. An awkward moment then arrives when the doctor announces, "I can't find anything wrong with you." The patient responds, "Then why do I feel so lousy all the time?" The answer is that there are probably a lot of reasons, which may include bad eating habits, poor self-image, boredom, frustrations with children, job dissatisfaction, lack of exercise and a troubled marriage.

Unfortunately, tackling such issues is no small project. The disease-oriented physician may reach for the prescription pad and supply a drug to dull the anxiety level or ship the patient to a psychiatrist, while muttering to himself that he'd prefer taking care of people who are "really sick." (Unfortunately, the patient in front of him probably will be really sick before long.) The physician who actively tries to deal with some of the complexities of the patient's lifestyle may have little more success than his fire-fighting colleague. For one thing, the patient may actually be disappointed to hear that there is no disease to account for the symptoms. A patient's comment that "there must be something you haven't found yet" may trigger a more expensive round of tests or perhaps an equally costly second opinion. This is especially likely in urban areas, where a missed diagnosis may result in a malpractice suit. Diagnostic tests which are ordered partly or wholly to avoid a losing battle with the legal profession account for a respectable portion of the nation's medical bills.

Even if the patient welcomes the reassurance that no serious pathology is apparent, bringing about meaningful changes in habits and attitudes may prove to be a formidable task. The doctor can describe the risks of smoking in sickening detail or rhapsodize on the benefits of quitting, but he or she cannot follow the patients around to extinguish their cigarettes. We know of no medical office which conducts pantry patrol or operates a shuttle service to Weight Watchers meetings. A physician cannot force anyone to start exercising, stop drinking, communicate better with spouse and kids, turn off the television or set some goals. (Frankly, many doctors have as big problems in these areas as their patients.)

For doctor and patient alike, perhaps the greatest obstacle to improving health is what Pastor Eugene H. Peterson describes as the "assumption that anything worthwhile can be acquired at once." In his thoughtful book *A Long Obedience in the Same Direction*, Peterson notes: "We assume that if something can be done at all, it can be done quickly and efficiently. Our attention spans have been conditioned by thirty-second commercials. Our sense of reality has been flattened by thirty-page abridgements."[4]

We forget too quickly that meaningful changes in lifestyle require a "long obedience": hundreds of small decisions made over a period of months and years. Most of these entail some degree of self-discipline or temporary self-denial, commodities which are rarely prized in an "instant society" (as Peterson calls it). "If it feels good, do it" has become a cliché, and too many of us continue to build our lives on the shifting sand of momentary feelings. Indeed, most of the plagues of the 1980s—including coronary disease, obesity, chemical dependency and sexually transmitted disease—are but the end point of day-to-day choices based on transient emotions.

In summary, most of Western medicine's practitioners, delivery systems and patients remain fixated on crisis care. As a society we seem more interested in putting out fires than in preventing them. We hope for technological solutions to our health problems while paying scant attention to the daily decisions which truly influence health. This behavior is on a collision course with its own price tag. The cost of all medical services, supplies and drugs is approaching the staggering level of three hundred billion dollars per year (about ten per cent of the gross national product) in the United States. As a result, lawmakers and insurance companies alike are scrambling to find ways to contain the spiraling costs of medical care. So far, though, the solutions have focused only on changing the flow of dollars and services: paying less for the same care (through "preferred provider" agreements in which insurance companies direct patients to physicians who accept lower fees), curtailing benefits (the current strategy of Medicare and Medicaid) and creating systems in which physicians assume some financial risk for the care provided (health maintenance organizations, or HMOs, which do not always live up to their title).

While Western medicine grapples with its priorities, the holistic health movement continues to proclaim a lofty vision of a New Medicine for a New Age. Unfortunately, as we have already described at some length, the movement's vanguard has managed to misdirect thousands of well-intentioned followers.

While criticizing overspecialization and lack of coordinated patient care by physicians, the holistic movement has cultivated a wildly diverse collection of alternative therapies which lack a common frame of reference. While reprimanding physicians for being rigid and authoritarian, many practitioners in the New Medicine have promoted their therapies with an evangelistic fervor, resisting independent confirmation of results.

While proclaiming the importance of individual responsibility for health, the holistic movement has provided ample opportunity for a passive "do something to me" mentality to flourish. Massage and manipulation, psychic healing and the various energy therapies all assume that something (visible or otherwise) needs to be done to or for the patient. Herbal concoctions, homeopathic remedies and unusual diets easily can assume the role of a magic potion.

Above all, the holistic health movement has served as a platform for disseminating the world view of the New Consciousness and promoting occultism as an approach to health.

Hope Remains

Those who seek to prevent lifestyle-related illness and promote wellness without embroiling themselves in Eastern mysticism and occultism should be encouraged, however, to know that there are a growing number of resources available to them. The majority of these are self-help books, but there are also some promising activities in the health-care field as well.

Some of the most sophisticated programs in whole-person care have been developed by the Wholistic Health Centers, headquartered in Hinsdale, Illinois. Founded over ten years ago by Dr. Granger Westberg, a clergyman with exceptional vision, the centers have pioneered an innovative, team-oriented approach to health care. Westberg first spearheaded the formation of a church-based clinic in Springfield, Ohio. The clinic's approach was unique: pastoral counselors and volunteer medical professionals worked in teams with patients to explore the role of lifestyle, stress and emotional problems in physical disease. The success of this concept led in 1973 to the establishment of the first Wholistic Health Center, which used church facilities in the affluent Chicago suburb of Hinsdale. One year later a second center opened in the rural community of Rockbridge, Illinois, and by 1982 a dozen centers were in operation in the Midwest and East.

A person seeking help at a center participates first in a health planning conference with a nurse, a physician and a pastor or psychologist. Here problems are defined, discussed and clarified, and then a treatment plan is formulated with a strong emphasis on the patient's responsibilities. Modalities of treatment include standard medical care, personal and family counseling and educational programs on a variety of subjects. Traditional, Western medicine is used but integrated into a much broader scope of care. New Consciousness mysticism and occultism are conspicuously absent.

The history, philosophy and approaches of the Wholistic Health Centers are nicely presented in the book *Wholistic Health* by Donald A. Tubesing.[5] Other publications, including the *Handbook of the Wholistic Medical Practice* and *44 Steps: The Complete Development Guide for Wholistic Health Care*, are valuable resources for health providers who desire to expand the horizons of their care. A quarterly journal, *Wholistic Wellspring*, contains worthwhile updates and perspectives as well.[6]

Another encouraging recent development has been the participation of hospitals in promoting wellness. For years, many hospitals have sponsored health fairs stressing early detection of disease through blood pressure screening, glaucoma checks and laboratory tests at nominal fees. More comprehensive programs centering on education for employees or the community at large are now becoming commonplace. The American Hospital Association's Center for Health Promotion has, since its inception in 1978, played a vigorous role in stimulating and assisting such programs. The Center now organizes a yearly Innovator's Conference, by invitation only, for pooling knowledge and generating new ideas.

Health promotion has also been initiated in business settings. Many corporations promote physical fitness among employees by sponsoring team sports or providing exercise equipment at the office or plant. One company, Western Federal Savings of Denver, has gone even further by developing a wellness education program for its employees. There are also plans for a comprehensive training curriculum in the near future. The idea of communicating basic health concepts through structured programs at the workplace has tremendous potential.[7] The fact that a wellness program is carried out by a hospital or a corporation does not, of course, guarantee the soundness of the ideas presented. Nevertheless, the vast majority of these have been grounded on straightforward, well-documented principles which are relatively free of the New Consciousness world view.

For those pursuing the subject of health at the local bookstore, there is no shortage of titles, particularly on the subjects of nutrition, weight reduction, exercise and the self-treatment of minor problems. Knowing where to begin a self-education project may prove difficult, however, because of the abundance of material which is of questionable value or grossly misleading. For those seeking guidance we have selected a few particularly useful volumes on specific subjects (such as nutrition or chronic fatigue) and listed them with annotations in the appendix.

11
The Biblical Foundation for Wholeness

UP TO THIS POINT we have invoked the teachings of the Old and New Testaments as a basis for critiquing the holistic health movement and warning of the hazards of tampering with the psychic realm. Scripture, of course, has much more to say about the human condition. In fact, the Bible provides a solid foundation and a wealth of insight for approaching the person who is ill, for preventing illness, and for creating the kind of balanced, enriched life which is the essence of wellness.

Biblical Wholeness
First, Scripture declares our significance as individuals created and loved by a sovereign God. David wrote,

O Lord, you have searched me and you know me.
You know when I sit and when I rise;
    you perceive my thoughts from afar.

You discern my going out and my lying down;
   you are familiar with all my ways.

For you created my inmost being;
   you knit me together in my mother's womb.
I praise you because I am fearfully and wonderfully made.
   (Ps 139:1-3, 13-14)

The very cornerstone of caring for ourselves and each other is this awareness of our worth, our importance as individuals. James Dobson has warned of the consequences of the contemporary "epidemic of inferiority" in his book *Hide or Seek:*

> Whenever the keys to self-esteem are seemingly out of reach for a large percentage of the people, as in twentieth-century America, then widespread "mental illness," neuroticism, hatred, alcoholism, drug abuse, violence, and social disorder will certainly occur. Personal worth is not something human beings are free to take or leave.[1]

There is ultimately no more secure basis for self-esteem than a working knowledge of this personal recognition by our Creator.

Second, Scripture orients us to the fallenness of humanity and the biological world. Even if we treat our bodies impeccably, they still eventually wear out and die. Unavoidable accidents, injuries, infections and genetic mistakes happen in the lives of the wise and foolish alike. "The whole creation has been groaning," wrote the apostle Paul, "as in the pains of childbirth right up to the present time. Not only so, but we ourselves . . . groan inwardly as we wait eagerly for . . . the redemption of our bodies" (Rom 8:22-23).

Not only does this help us deal both with annoyances and catastrophes, but it also helps us understand that achieving anything of value—including good health—is an uphill struggle. Without deliberate effort and maintenance, muscles become weak, fat accumulates, teeth decay, marriages crumble, and the mind stagnates. Once we have realized that this tendency toward deterioration in ourselves and disorder in our relationships is a universal pattern in the fallen world, we can avoid wallowing in self-pity and get on with constructive activity.

Third, Scripture makes it abundantly clear that we have a personal responsibility for excellence in our physical condition, our thinking, our behavior and our relationships. Paul wrote that the body is "meant . . . for the Lord, and the Lord for the body" (1 Cor 6:13). For the believer in Christ the issue is not only that of God's ownership of our lives, but the very presence of Christ in the believer. This puts an entirely new perspective on our conduct. Paul invoked this fact as a powerful argument against sexual promiscuity:

> Do you not know that your bodies are members of Christ himself? Shall I then take the members of Christ and unite them with a prostitute? Never! . . .
>
> Flee from sexual immorality. All other sins a man commits are outside his body, but he who sins sexually sins against his own body. Do you not know that your body is a temple of the Holy Spirit, who is in you, whom you have received from God? You are not your own; you were bought at a price. Therefore, honor God with your body. (1 Cor 6:15, 18-20)

Likewise, there is no more succinct statement on monitoring what we allow to enter and dwell in our minds than the exhortation that "whatever is right, whatever is pure, whatever is lovely, whatever is admirable—if anything is excellent or praiseworthy—think about such things" (Phil 4:8).

Fourth, Scripture reminds us of our limitations. Though wisdom and health are much to be desired, they are not ends in themselves. Apart from being rightly related to God, they are pointless. In Ecclesiastes King Solomon surveyed his wisdom, pleasures and accomplishments—which were legendary in the ancient world, as they are now—and declared in no uncertain terms that they were meaningless, a "chasing after the wind" (Eccles 1:14). "Here is the conclusion of the matter," he wrote. "Fear God and keep his commandments, for this is the whole duty of man" (Eccles 12:13).

Scriptural Counsel
Aside from orienting our thinking and ordering our priorities,

the Bible contains valuable encouragement and advice for the sick and the well alike.

For those who are ill, there are words of comfort: affliction will ultimately end, and while present it can be an occasion both for learning compassion and gaining inner strength. Paul reminded the Corinthian church that "the Father of compassion . . . comforts us in all our troubles, so that we can comfort those in any trouble with the comfort we ourselves have received from God" (2 Cor 1:3-4). In addition to the harassment and indignities which he suffered at the hands of his adversaries, Paul also endured a "thorn in the flesh" which many commentators believe was a physical ailment. God's response to his repeated prayers that the suffering be relieved was this: "My grace is sufficient for you, for my power is made perfect in weakness" (2 Cor 12:8).

For those who seek to prevent illness, there are numerous guidelines for temperate behavior. Indeed, if the human race would tomorrow begin to abide by biblical standards, we would see a revolution in health. There would be an end to the physical deterioration, violence and accidents which result from alcohol abuse (with a saving of over twenty-five thousand lives every year from drunk-driving accidents alone). Self-destruction from illicit drug use would cease. The current epidemic of sexually transmitted disease would come to an end. The incalculable physical and social effects of anxiety, hatred, loneliness and disrupted relationships would disappear. S. I. McMillen offers a detailed and highly readable description of these benefits and of the Old Testament sanitation guidelines which, when practiced, prevented illness and death among the Israelites. His book None of These Diseases is a classic.[2]

For those who desire wellness, Scripture offers even more than prevention of the physical and mental illnesses caused by violating God's standards of behavior. The result of living under the control of the Holy Spirit, we are told, is no less than the most optimal state of emotional health: "But the fruit of the Spirit is love, joy, peace, patience, kindness, goodness, faithfulness, gentleness and self-control" (Gal 5:22). The by-product of continuously communicating our needs and desires to God is an inner tranquility "which transcends all understanding" (Phil 4:7). The teachings of Jesus on worry are familiar but have been forgotten by a society in which anxiety seems to have become a national state of mind:

> Therefore I tell you, do not worry about your life, what you will eat or drink; or about your body, what you will wear. Is not life more important than food, and the body more important than clothes? Look at the birds of the air; they do not sow or reap or store away in barns, and yet your heavenly Father feeds them. Are you not much more valuable than they? Who of you by worrying can add a single hour to his life? (Mt 6:25-27)

Beyond even physical and emotional health, God offers the security of knowing our ultimate destination if we will abandon our willfulness and submit to his authority. Furthermore, in exchange for the stagnation and despair which stems from preoccupation with self, God offers the enormous satisfaction of being his representative on earth and participating in changing the lives of others.

Because the world "groans" and is fallen, we are not offered any guarantee of freedom from illness, adversity and danger during our stay on earth. We are promised that, if we have accepted God's pardon for our fallenness and rebellion—the pardon which is available only because Jesus Christ suffered and died in our place—our final destiny will include that freedom and much more. In the meantime, we are offered the ultimate resource—God himself—for making the most of our lives, regardless of circumstances. Writing from prison, the apostle Paul declared:

> I know what it is to be in need, and I know what it is to have plenty. I have learned the secret of being content in any and every situation, whether well fed or hungry, whether living in plenty or in want. I can do everything through him who gives me strength. (Phil 4:12-13)

One need not look for a better definition of wholeness.

Appendix:
Recommended Books for Those in Pursuit of Wellness

Inner Energy by M. F. Graham, M.D. New York: Sterling Publishing, 1978.
This is arguably the best book available for the person combating chronic fatigue. Both detailed and readable, it covers a gamut of factors ranging from pathological disease to diet, exercise and goal setting. At least one-half of the adults visiting any primary-care physician would benefit enormously from careful digestion of Graham's suggestions.

The Aerobics Way by Kenneth Cooper, M.D. New York: M. Evans and Co., 1977.
There are now many books on the market extolling running and other forms of aerobic exercise (exercise in which higher levels of oxygen are consumed, such as jogging, swimming, cycling), but Dr. Cooper was a prime mover in putting aerobics on the map in the early 1970s. This follow-up to his earlier books (*Aerobics*, *The New Aerobics* and *Aerobics for Women*, written with Mrs. Cooper) presents an excellent discussion of the risk factors for coronary artery disease. It also includes updated charts which al-

low one to become gradually conditioned in any of several aerobic activities. Cooper's Aerobics Center in Dallas is worth the trip.

Take Care of Yourself: A Consumer's Guide to Medical Care by Donald M. Vickery, M.D., and James F. Fries, M.D. Reading, Mass.: Addison-Wesley, 1976.

The Medicine Show, Rev., by the editors of *Consumer Reports.* Mount Vernon, N. Y.: Pantheon Books, Random House, 1980.

These volumes are excellent resources for those who wish to prevent unnecessary trips to the doctor or improper use of home remedies. The first features simple flow charts for dozens of common problems. These charts greatly simplify one's decision process. The second book covers much the same ground, but adds *Consumer Reports'* well-known jaundiced view of useless or overpriced medications. Other health books by Consumer Union (such as *Health Quackery*) are well researched and fair, as are the occasional articles on medications in *Consumer Reports.*

Jane Brody's Nutrition Book by Jane Brody. New York: W. W. Norton, 1981.

The Complete Food Handbook by Roger P. Doyle and James L. Redding. New York: Grove Press, 1976.

Wholesome Diet by the editors of Time-Life Books. New York: Time-Life Books, 1981.

There appears to be no end in sight to the flow of books designed to help us lose weight, eat right and avoid the ravages of additives, sugar and "toxins." The above books are noteworthy for their restraint in a field in which misinformation, mythology and poor documentation abound. *Jane Brody's Nutrition Book,* by the prolific health columnist of the *New York Times,* is notable for its comprehensive and well-researched information. Topics covered include the basics of nutrients, obesity and weight control, special diets and the role of vitamins and additives. *The Complete Food Handbook* takes food in groups and quite fairly considers issues such as preservatives, "organic" foods and vitamins. Its authors are not afraid to be hard on both the food industry and the health-food set alike. *Wholesome Diet* is one of several excellent volumes in the Time-Life Library of Health, which also includes books on cancer, heart disease, headache and the common cold. All are graced by an interesting text, superb illustrations and sensible information.

None of These Diseases by S. I. McMillen, M.D. Old Tappan, N. J.: Revell, 1963.

Happiness Is a Choice by Frank B. Minirth, M.D., and Paul D. Meier, M.D. Grand Rapids, Mich.: Baker Book House, 1978.

There's a Lot More to Health Than Not Being Sick by Bruce Larson. Waco,
  Tex.: Word Books, 1981.

When I Relax, I Feel Guilty by Tim Hansel. Elgin, Ill.: David C. Cook, 1979.

These books explore various components of lifestyle. McMillen's book is
somewhat of a classic, showing how well the Scriptures tie in with modern
medical knowledge. (For example, the ceremonial washings of the Hebrews prevented the spread of infectious disease.) *Happiness Is a Choice*
is a comprehensive manual on depression written by psychiatrists who are
also assistant professors in the Pastoral Ministries Department of Dallas
Theological Seminary. Bruce Larson's book deals with basic themes such
as friendship, hope and responsibility, and their role in preserving health.
When I Relax, I Feel Guilty, despite its misleadingly cute title and cover, is
as powerful and profound a statement on living life to the fullest as can be
found anywhere. Hansel's suggestions on maxi- and mini-vacations are too
numerous to be digested in one sitting, and the entire book is worth several
readings.

Notes

Chapter 1: The Dawn of Holistic Health

[1]Harold J. Morowitz, "The Six Million Dollar Man," *Hospital Practice*, May 1977.

[2]Daniel Schorr, *Don't Get Sick in America* (Nashville, Tenn.: Aurora Publishers, 1970); Howard Lewis and Martha Lewis, *The Medical Offenders* (New York: Simon and Schuster, 1970); Sam McClatchie, *Misdirected Medicine* (New York: Walker and Co., 1973); Ivan Illich, *Medical Nemesis* (New York: Pantheon, 1976); Edgar Berman, M.D., *The Solid Gold Stethoscope* (New York: Macmillan, 1976).

[3]Leslie J. Kaslof, ed., *Wholistic Dimensions in Healing* (Garden City, N.Y.: Doubleday, 1978).

[4]Two examples: (1) Adelaid Bry with Marjorie Blair, "The Medicine of the Mind," *Cosmopolitan*, July 1978, pp. 169-71, 266. (Excerpted from the book *Directing the Movies of Your Mind* [New York: Harper and Row, 1978].) (2) Beverly Russell, "Energy Dynamics," *House and Garden*, July 1978, pp. 86, 164.

[5]Dennis M. Warren, "Legal Considerations in the Search for Holistic Health," in *Journal of Holistic Health* (San Diego: The Word Shop, 1978), p. 104.

Chapter 2: Ten Articles of Faith in the New Medicine

[1]George Leonard, "The Holistic Health Revolution," in *The Journal of Holistic Health* (San Diego: Assoc. for Holistic Health, 1977), p. 81.

[2]Richard Svihus, "The Concept of Holistic Health: Origins and Definitions," in *The Journal of Holistic Health* (San Diego: Assoc. for Holistic Health, 1977), p. 17.

[3]Ibid., p. 19.

[4]Rick Ingrasci, "Holistic Health," *New Age Magazine*, May 1978, p. 4.

[5]Amy Wallace and Bill Henkin, *The Psychic Healing Book* (New York: Delacorte Press, 1978), p. 64.

[6]A. M. C. G. Harvey et al. *The Principles and Practice of Medicine*, 20th ed. (New York: Appleton-Century-Crofts, 1980), pp. 1373-88.

[7]John F. Thie, *Touch for Health* (Marina del Rey, Calif.: DeVorss and Co., 1973), p. 6.

[8]Svihus, "The Concept of Holistic Health," p. 17.

[9]See, for example, Elmer and Alyce Green, *Beyond Biofeedback* (New York: Delacorte Press, 1977).

[10]For an example of Dr. Jensen's metaphysical outlook, see "Health and Spirituality: An Interview with Dr. Bernard Jensen," in *Rays from the Rose Cross*, May 1978, pp. 226-29. In this interview for the official journal of the Rosicrucian Society (a heavily mystical organization which he refers to as his "spiritual abode"), Dr. Jensen expounds on topics such as the divine nature of man and the value of astrologic diagnosis. Interestingly, in some views the iris seems to function as a contact point for psychic diagnosis of a patient's condition.

[11]Allie Simon, David M. Worthen, M.D., Lt. John A. Mitas, II, M.C., USN, "An Evaluation of Iridology," *Journal of the American Medical Association* 242 (28 Sept. 1979):1385-89.

[12]Harold H. Bloomfield and Robert B. Kory, *The Holistic Way to Health and Happiness* (New York: Simon and Schuster, 1978).

[12a]Edward R. Friedlander, "Dream Your Cancer Away: The Simontons" in Douglas Stalker and Clark Glymour (eds.) *Examining Holistic Medicine* (Buffalo, New York: Prometheus Books 1985) pp 273-87.

[13]Linda A. Clark, *Help Yourself to Health* (New York: Pyramid Books, 1972).

[14]For further information, see also John Weldon and Zola Levitt, *Psychic Healing* (Chicago: Moody Press, 1982).

[15]Quoted in Svihus, "The Concept of Holistic Health," p. 17.

[16]Arthur S. Freese, "Dr. Shealy and His New Medicine," in C. Norman Shealy, *Occult Medicine Can Save Your Life* (New York: Dial Press, 1975), p. 2.

[17]C. S. Lewis, *Poems* (New York: Harcourt Brace Jovanovich, 1964), p. 55.

[18]James Fadiman, "The Prime Cause of Healing," in *The Journal of Holistic Health* (San Diego: Assoc. for Holistic Health, 1977), pp. 13-14.

[19]Robert Gerard, "Integral Psychology and Esoteric Healing," in *Journal of Holistic Health* (San Diego: The Word Shop, 1979), pp. 34-35.

[20]Ibid., p. 34.

[21]A detailed analysis of the "death and dying" movement is available in John Weldon's book *Is There Life after Death?* (Irvine, Calif.: Harvest House, 1977). See also the excellent synopsis contained in the April 1977 *Journal of the Spiritual Conterfeits Project* (available from the Spiritual Counterfeits Project, P.O. Box 4308, Berkeley, CA 94704).

Chapter 3: Energy: The Common Denominator

[1]Mary Coddington, *In Search of the Healing Energy* (New York: Warner Books, 1978), p. 12.

[2]Quoted in ibid., p. 18.

[3]Irving Oyle, *Time, Space and the Mind* (Millbrae, Calif.: Celestial Arts, 1976), p. viii.

[4]Ibid.

[5]Ann Nietzke, "Portrait of an Aura Reader," *Human Behavior*, Feb. 1979, p. 31.

[6]Ibid., p. 31.

[7]William Tiller, "Creating a New Functional Model of Body Healing Energies," *Journal of Holistic Health* (San Diego: The Word Shop, 1978), p. 46.

[8]Quoted in Nietzke, "Portrait of an Aura Reader," p. 31.

[9]Evarts G. Loomis, "The Healing Center of the Future," in *The Journal of Holistic Health* (San Diego: Assoc. for Holistic Health, 1977), p. 73.

[10]Jack Gibb, "Psycho-Sociological Aspects of Holistic Health," in *The Journal of Holistic Health* (San Diego: Assoc. for Holistic Health, 1977), p. 44.

[11]The dangers of involvement with yogic practices are discussed in John Weldon's book *Occult Shock and Psychic Forces* (San Diego, Calif.: Master Books, 1980), pp. 72-78. Reprinted by Global Publishers.

[12]M. J. Nightingale, "Air and Light," in *A Visual Encyclopedia of Unconventional Medicine*, ed. Ann Hill (New York: Crown Publishers, 1979), p. 92.

[13]Quoted in Clark, *Help Yourself to Health*, p. 106.

[14]Coddington, *In Search of the Healing Energy*, pp. 140-41.

[15]Ken Dychtwald, "Sexuality and the Whole Person," in *The Holistic Health Handbook* (Berkeley, Calif.: And/Or Press, 1978), p. 304.

[16]Quoted in Nikhilananda, *Vivekananda: The Yogas and Other Works* (New York: Rama Krishna-Vivekananda Center, 1953), pp. 592-93, 598.

[17]D. Gareth Jones, *Our Fragile Brains* (Downers Grove, Ill.: InterVarsity

Press, 1981).

[18]Dolores Krieger, *The Therapeutic Touch: How to Use Your Hands to Help or Heal* (Englewood Cliffs, N.J.: Prentice-Hall, 1979), p. 13.

[19]Ibid., p. 13, emphasis added.

[20]Ibid., pp. 49-50.

[21]Ibid., p. 70.

[22]Ibid., p. 71.

[23]Ibid., p. 77.

[24]Ibid., p. 80.

[25]Fritjof Capra, *The Tao of Physics* (Boulder, Colo.: Shambhala Publications, 1976).

[26]We owe this summarizing of New Consciousness thinking to the excellent pamphlet *Occult Philosophy and Mystical Experience* by Brooks Alexander. This is well worth reading in its entirety and may be obtained from the Spiritual Counterfeits Project, P.O. Box 4308, Berkeley, CA 94704.

Chapter 4: The Mystical Roots

[1]Ilza Veith, trans., *Huang Ti Nei Ching Su Wen (The Yellow Emperor's Classic of Internal Medicine)* (Berkeley: Univ. of California Press, 1966), p. 4.

[2]Ibid., p. 10, emphasis added.

[3]Teruo Matsumoto, M.D., *Acupuncture for Physicians* (Springfield, Ill.: Charles C. Thomas, 1974), p. 3.

[4]Terence M. Murphy, M.D., and John J. Bonica, M.D., "Acupuncture Analgesia and Anesthesia," *Archives of Surgery* 112 (July 1977):898.

[5]Mary Austin, *Acupuncture Therapy* (New York: A.S.I. Publishers, 1972), p. 119.

Chapter 5: Acupuncture's Questionable Triumphs

[1]John J. Bonica, M.D., "Therapeutic Acupuncture in the People's Republic of China," *Journal of the American Medical Association* 228 (17 June 1974):1545.

[2]Peter Koenig, "The Americanization of Acupuncture," *Psychology Today*, June 1973, p. 37.

[3]Marc Duke, *Acupuncture* (New York: Pyramid Publications, 1972), p. 1.

[4]Bonica, "Therapeutic Acupuncture," p. 1548.

[5]Ibid., p. 1549, his emphasis.

[6]The following are samples of articles in the medical literature. They illustrate the variety of clinical situations and experimental designs which have been used in studying acupuncture.

a) A study of one hundred chronic pain patients (who had not improved with conventional treatments) at the University of Washington in 1976 found that patients showed spectacular improvement initially but disappointing long-term response. A few patients who claimed to feel better for a longer period were found to be taking no less medication and demonstrating no functional improvement. (T. M. Murphy, "Subjective and Objective Follow-up Assessment of Acupuncture Therapy," in J. J. Bonica and D. Albe-Fessard, eds., *Advances in Pain Research and Therapy* (New York: Raven Press, 1976), pp. 811-15.

b) A study (also at the University of Washington in 1976) of tooth pain induced in volunteers using electrical current showed a significant response to acupuncture. It was noted that acupuncture needles applied to intrasegmental areas of skin—that is, those whose nerves connect to the same level of the spinal cord as the nerves supplying the teeth—produced much more effective pain relief than needles inserted at distant parts of the body. (C. R. Chapman et al., "Effects of Intrasegmental Electrical Acupuncture on Dental Pain: Evaluation by Threshold Estimation and Sensory Decision Theory," *Pain* 3 [1977]:213-27.)

c) Forty-two patients with chronic shoulder pain were treated at Temple University in 1974. Half received acupuncture and half a procedure in which the skin was lightly touched but not penetrated. All patients reported subjective improvement. Patients were also tested for susceptibility to hypnosis; those who showed little or no susceptibility tended to experience lower levels of relief. (Mary E. Moore and Stephen N. Berk, "Acupuncture for Chronic Shoulder Pain," *Annals of Internal Medicine* 84 [1976]:381-84.)

d) Investigators at the University of California at San Francisco studied a small group of thirty-seven patients who were treated for problems including migraine headache, neck and back pain, bursitis in various locations, painful menstruation, and pain associated with nerve damage. Acupuncture was found to produce at least temporary relief in most of the patients with chronic pain, permanent relief in some cases of acute pain (such as menstrual cramps), and little improvement where nerve damage was present (for example, in an amputated limb). Patients who scored highly on tests of anxiety and depression, as well as those with good doctor-patient rapport, experienced more impressive pain relief. (J. D. Levin, J. Gormley, and Howard L. Fields, "Observations on the Analgesic Effects of Needle Puncture," *Pain* 2 [1976]:149-59.)

e) Forty patients with degenerative arthritis affecting various joints were treated at the New England Medical Center Hospital using either traditional acupuncture points or nearby control points. Both groups showed significant improvements in pain and tenderness, lasting at least six weeks after eight treatments, with no significant difference between groups. (A. C. Shaw, L. W. Chang, and L. Shaw, "Efficacy of Acupuncture on Osteoarthritic Pain," *New England Journal of Medicine* 293

[1975]:375-78.)

f) In a large collection of patients (261) with a wide variety of pain disorders, physicians at the University of Florida noted three characteristics of response to acupuncture. First, there appeared to be no difference in pain relief between needling of classical points and of arbitrary points at a distance. Second, regardless of location of needling, significantly higher numbers of patients reported increased pain relief with repeated treatments (a total of four were given). Third, for a large number of patients there was a recurrence of pain within four weeks of the last treatment. (P. K. Lee et al., "Treatment of Chronic Pain with Acupuncture," *Journal of the American Medical Association* 232 [16 June 1975]:1133-35.)

[7]R. Melzack, D. Stillwell, and E. Fox, "Trigger Points and Acupuncture Points for Pain: Correlations and Implications," *Pain* 3 [1977]:3-23.

[8]Ronald Melzack, "How Acupuncture Works: A Sophisticated Western Theory Takes the Mystery Out," *Psychology Today*, June 1973, p. 34.

[9]Thie, *Touch for Health*, p. 16.

[10]Felix Mann, M.D., *Acupuncture* (New York: Vintage Books, 1973), p. 5.

[11]Ibid., p. 228.

[12]Sheila Ostrander and Lynn Schroeder, *Psychic Discoveries behind the Iron Curtain* (Englewood Cliffs, N. J.: Prentice-Hall, 1970), p. 227.

[13]Ibid., p. 230.

[14]Thelma Moss, *The Probability of the Impossible* (Los Angeles: J. P. Tarcher, 1974).

[15]Mann, *Acupuncture*, p. 229.

[16]Ibid., p. 230.

Chapter 6: The Popular Therapies

[1]Thie, *Touch for Health*, p. 6.

[2]Ibid., p. 10.

[3]Ibid., p. 12.

[4]Ibid., p. 16, emphasis added.

[5]Clive Johnson, "Touch for Health," *Science of Mind*, Sept. 1977, p. 99.

[6]John Diamond, M.D., *Behavioral Kinesiology* (New York: Harper and Row, 1979), p. 28.

[7]Ibid., p. 21.

[8]Ibid.

[9]Ibid., p. 107.

[10]Ibid., p. 114.

[11]Walter Fischman and Mark Grinims, "The Muscle Response Test," *Family Circle*, 20 Feb. 1979, p. 113.

[12]Iona Teeguarden, *Acupressure Way of Health: Jin Shin Do* (Tokyo: Japan Publications, 1978), p. 9.

[13]Ibid., p. 14.
[14]Ibid., p. 21.
[15]Ibid., pp. 31-32.
[16]Ibid., p. 27.
[17]Ibid., p. 156.
[18]Dr. Motoyama is founder and director of the International Association for Religion and Parapsychology and is credited with developing instrumentation to measure meridians and "subtle energies of the body."
[19]Brooks Alexander, "Holistic Health from the Inside," *Journal of the Spiritual Counterfeits Project*, Aug. 1978, p. 16.

Chapter 7: A Sampling of Psychics

[1]Ambrose A. Worrall and Olga N. Worrall, *The Gift of Healing* (New York: Harper and Row, 1965); Worrall and Worrall, *Explore Your Psychic World* (New York: Harper and Row, 1970).
[2]Worrall and Worrall, *The Gift of Healing*, p. 187.
[3]W. Brugh Joy, *Joy's Way* (Los Angeles: J. P. Tarcher, 1979), pp. 206-7.
[4]Ibid., p. 7.
[5]Lawrence LeShan, *The Medium, the Mystic, and the Physicist* (New York: Ballantine, 1974), p. 86.
[6]Ibid., p. 87.
[7]Ibid., p. 102.
[8]Ibid., p. 106.
[9]Ibid., p. 107.
[10]Ibid., p. 110.
[11]Ibid., p. 117.
[12]John G. Fuller, *Arigo: Surgeon of the Rusty Knife* (New York: Thomas Y. Crowell, 1974), pp. 18-19.
[13]Ibid., p. 108.
[14]Ibid., p. 238.
[15]Thomas Sugrue, *There Is a River* (New York: Holt, Rinehart and Winston, 1942), pp. 166-67.
[16]Ibid., p. 47.
[17]Ibid., p. 107.
[18]Ibid., p. 112.
[19]Ibid., p. 204.
[20]Ibid., p. 210.
[21]Ibid., p. 304.
[22]Hugh Lynn Cayce, *Venture Inward* (New York: Harper and Row, 1964), p. 11.
[23]We would love to take credit for this play on words, but it was borrowed from Gary North's excellent review of Edgar Cayce in *None Dare Call It*

Witchcraft (Westport, Conn.: Arlington House Pub., 1976).

²⁴Thomas Sugrue, *Stranger in the Earth* (New York: Holt, Rinehart and Winston, 1948), pp. 215-16.

²⁵Sugrue, *There Is a River*, p. 350.

²⁶Reilly's work with Cayce and current recommendations for healthy living are compiled in *The Edgar Cayce Handbook for Health through Drugless Therapy* (New York: Macmillan, 1975).

²⁷William A. McGarey, M.D., *Edgar Cayce and the Palma Christi*, 2 vols. (Virginia Beach: A.R.E. Press, n.d.).

²⁸Reilly, *Edgar Cayce Handbook*, p. xviii.

²⁹Sugrue, *There Is a River*, pp. 323-24.

³⁰William A. McGarey, M.D., "Applying Edgar Cayce Readings to the Daily Clinical Practice of Medicine," in *Journal of Holistic Health* (San Diego: Mandala Society, 1975), p. 49.

³¹Ibid.

³²Ibid., p. 50.

Chapter 8: A Check List for Your Neighborhood Healer

¹Norman Cousins, *Anatomy of an Illness As Perceived by the Patient* (New York: W. W. Norton, 1979).

²(Philadelphia: Saunders, 1966).

³O. Carl Simonton, M.D., Stephanie Matthews-Simonton, and James Creighton, *Getting Well Again* (Los Angeles: J. P. Tarcher, 1978).

⁴For some excellent observations on this practice, see Stanley Dokupil, "Seizing the Power: The Use of Imagination for Healing," *Spiritual Counterfeits Project Newsletter*, Oct.-Nov. 1982, pp. 1-4.

⁵William A. Nolen, M.D., *Healing: A Doctor in Search of a Miracle* (New York: Random House, 1974).

⁶Ibid., p. 308.

⁷Fuller, *Arigo*, p. 134.

⁸James W. Sire, *The Universe Next Door* (Downers Grove, Ill.: InterVarsity Press, 1976).

⁹The dangers (physical, mental and spiritual) of involvement in occultism and the psychic realm are discussed in detail in John Weldon's book *The Hazards of Psychic Involvement: A Look at the Consequences* (unpublished), as well as in Kurt Koch's classic *Occult Bondage and Deliverance* (Grand Rapids, Mich.: Kregel Publications, 1970).

Chapter 9 Examining Controversial Therapies

¹One thorny problem related to sincere providers of questionable therapies is raised by the practice of chiropractic, a subject discussed briefly elsewhere in this volume. Many evangelicals use or accept chiro-

practic, some are chiropractors themselves, and few would consider this form of therapy to be unorthodox. Yet despite its widespread acceptance this practice has a somewhat checkered history, and the basic suppositions of D.D. Palmer (regarding "subluxations" of the spine as a cause of numberous bodily ailments) have been challenged for decades. (See, for example, W. Jarvis " Chiropractic" in *The Skeptical Inquirer* (Fall 1987); Edmund S. Crelin, "Chiropractic," in D. Stalker and C. Glymour, *Examining Holistic Medicine* (Prometheus Books, 1985); R.L. Smith, *At Your Own Risk: The Case Against Chiropractic* (Pocket Books 1959); the editors of Consumers Union, "Chiropractors, Healers or Quacks?" in Consumers Union, *Health Quackery* (Holt Rinehart and Winston, 1980).)

On the other hand, many chiropractors are making a concerted effort to subject their therapies to scientific scrutiny, and are not necessarily accepting the subluxation theory as an legitimate explanantion for successful results. Many health practices, both past and present, have proved beneficial even with faulty reasoning. Within a field as widespread as chiropractic, there are certainly those who practice wisely and within defined limits, and also those who make exaggerated claims and mislead (or even injure) many.

For the record, Mr. Weldon urges that the critical literature cited above (as well has his own material on chiropractic in C. Wilson and J. Weldon, *Psychic Forces* (Global Publishers, 1987), pp. 204-217) be read, and the arguments therein be weighed carefully, before beginning or continuing treatment.

Chapter 10: Alternatives to the New Medicine

[1]Shealy, *Occult Medicine Can Save Your Life*, p. 168, Shealy's emphasis.

[2]Rene Dúbos, *Mirage of Health* (New York: Harper and Row, 1959).

[3]Thomas McKeown, *The Role of Medicine: Dream, Mirage, or Nemesis?* (London: Nullfield Provincial Hospitals Trust, 1976).

[4]Eugene Peterson, *A Long Obedience in the Same Direction* (Downers Grove, Ill.: InterVarsity Press, 1980), pp. 11-12.

[5]Donald Tubesing, *Wholistic Health: A Whole-Person Approach to Primary Health Care* (New York: Human Sciences Press, 1979).

[6]These materials may be obtained by writing to Wholistic Health Centers, Inc., 137 S. Garfield Ave., Hinsdale, IL 60521.

[7]A number of programs are summarized in the book *14 Days to a Wellness Lifestyle* by Donald Ardell (Mill Valley, Calif.: Whatever Publishing, 1982).

Chapter 11: The Biblical Foundation for Wholeness

[1]James Dobson, *Hide or Seek* (Old Tappan, N. J.: Revell, 1979), pp. 20-21.

[2]S. I. McMillen, *None of These Diseases* (Old Tappan, N.J.: Revell, 1963).

Bibliography

This listing is highly selective (based on general importance or our own interest) and annotated with our personal evaluations. A book's presence here does not imply endorsement.

Anthologies
Albright, Peter, and Albright, Bets Parker, eds. *Body, Mind, and Spirit: The Journey toward Health and Wholeness.* Brattleboro, Vt.: Stephen Greene Press, 1980.

Carlson, Rick J., ed. *The Frontiers of Science and Medicine.* Chicago: Henry Regnery Company, 1975.

Flynn, Patricia Anne Randolph, ed. *The Healing Continuum: Journeys in the Philosophy of Holistic Health.* Bowie, Md.: Robert J. Brady Company, 1980.

Goldwag, Elliott M., ed. *Inner Balance: The Power of Holistic Healing.* Englewood Cliffs, N. J.: Prentice-Hall, 1979.

Hastings, Arthur C.; Fadiman, James; and Gordon, James S., eds. *Health for the Whole Person.* Boulder, Colo.: Westview Press, 1980.

Otto, Herbert, and Knight, James W., eds. *Dimensions in Wholistic Healing: New Frontiers in the Treatment of the Whole Person.* Chicago: Nelson-Hall, 1979.

Sobel, David S., ed. *Ways of Health: Holistic Approaches to Ancient and Contemporary Medicine*. New York: Harcourt Brace Jovanovich, 1979. All of the above books contain selections of articles relating to holistic health with a strong slant toward the New Consciousness world view. The most coherent of these is *Health for the Whole Person*, which contains some interesting perspectives mixed in with plenty of mysticism. It also features an introduction by Senator Edward Kennedy and extensive annotated bibliographies after each chapter.

Handbooks and Guidebooks

Association for Holistic Health. *Journal of Holistic Health*. This yearly offering contains transcriptions from the previous year's conference of the Association for Holistic Health (and the Mandala Society) in San Diego. These are extremely interesting for those who wish to keep up with current trends in the holistic health movement. The conferences traditionally have featured strong doses of New Consciousness. Available from Mandala Open Circle, P.O. Box 1233, Del Mar, CA 92014.

Berkeley Holistic Health Center. *The Holistic Health Handbook*. Berkeley, Calif.: And/Or Press, 1978. An anthology of techniques which strongly leans toward the various alternative therapies of the New Medicine. Very comprehensive and laced with New Consciousness thinking.

Kaslof, Leslie J. *Wholistic Dimensions in Healing: A Resource Guide*. Garden City, N. Y.: Doubleday and Company, 1978. This guidebook consists primarily of resources for various alternative therapies. Within any given specialty are listed researchers, therapists, journals and centers, all with brief descriptions. Heavy leaning toward New-Age resources.

Kulvinskas, Victoras. *Survival into the 21st Century*. Wethersfield, Conn.: Omangod Press, 1975. Subtitled "Planetary Healers Manual," this guidebook looks somewhat like a remnant from commune days in the late 1960s. Lots of New-Age nutrition mixed with yoga and other assorted topics.

Lande, Nathaniel. *Mindstyles/Lifestyles*. Los Angeles: Price/Stern/Sloan Publishers, 1976. This is extremely useful for anyone who wishes a capsule summary of dozens of philosophies and lifestyles. Lande has not left a stone unturned. Very instructive as a survey of the places one can look to "find oneself" in today's popular philosophy market.

Penzer, Mark, ed. *The Journal of Energy Medicine*. This very slick and expensive journal contains every imaginable viewpoint in medicine, orthodox and alternative. Some interesting material and professional graphics.

De Smedt, Evelyn, et al. *Lifearts*. New York: St. Martin's Press, 1977. This stresses the world views of the ancients as applied to nutrition, healing, sex and nature. Originally from France.

General Surveys of the Holistic Health Movement

Bloomfield, Harold H., and Kory, Robert B. *The Holistic Way to Health and Happiness*. New York: Simon and Schuster, 1978. This book soft-pedals mysticism, although it contains many references to the value of Transcendental Meditation. (Bloomfield is a TM initiator.) It stresses general lifestyle improvement, stress reduction and elimination of bad habits such as smoking. It is also a classic example of the use of a slick presentation to make a mystical or occult product attractive to the unwary seeker of "health and happiness."

Hill, Ann, ed. *A Visual Encyclopedia of Unconventional Medicine*. Great Britain: Triune Books Ltd., 1978. A comprehensive introduction to the spectrum of alternative health practices. Lots of pictures and graphics and a heavy New Consciousness slant.

Kingston, Jeremy. *Healing without Medicine*. London: Aldus Books Ltd., 1975. One of a series of picture books on the supernatural with a survey attitude rather than a particular spiritual viewpoint.

Oyle, Irving. *The Healing Mind*. Millbrae, Calif.: Celestial Arts, 1975.

——————. *Magic, Mysticism, and Modern Medicine: Journal of a Family Physician*. Millbrae, Calif.: Celestial Arts, 1976.

——————. *Time, Space, and the Mind*. Millbrae, Calif.: Celestial Arts, 1976.

——————. *The New American Medicine Show*. Santa Cruz, Calif.: Unity Press, 1979.

These books by Dr. Oyle contain everything from incisive prose to free association. Very heavy on the "we are all energy" theme, but rarely dull. Recommended for those who wish to understand a full-blown New Consciousness mindset toward healing.

Popenoe, Cris. *Wellness*. Washington, D.C.: Yes! Inc., 1977. This is the ultimate annotated bibliography, organized by subject matter. As usual, a heavy slant toward the alternative therapies, life energies and so on.

Shealy, C. Norman. *Occult Medicine Can Save Your Life*. New York: Dial Press, 1975. A general introduction to the New Medicine. Some interesting personal accounts mixed with uncritical embracing of everything from astrology to aura reading. Most writers in the holistic health movement love the book but hate the title: occultism has too many negative connotations, but Dr. Shealy is at least up front about the sources of many alternative therapies.

Specialties in the New Medicine

Benson, Herbert. *The Relaxation Response*. New York: Avon Books, 1975.

A genuine effort to demystify the effects of meditation on the body. Benson studied practitioners of Transcendental Meditation at Harvard Medical School and came up with his own nonreligious approach to relaxation and stress reduction.

Bricklin, Mark. *The Practical Encyclopedia of Natural Healing.* Emmaus, Penn.: Rodale Press, 1976. How to cure everything from acne to warts using natural therapies (mostly vitamins and minerals), by the executive editor of *Prevention* magazine. Contains endorsements of acupuncture, reflexology and yoga, among others, mixed in with the nutritional suggestions. Credit is due this volume for backing some of its dietary advice with documented studies and not merely anecdotes.

Brown, Barbara B. *Stress and the Art of Biofeedback.* New York: Harper and Row, 1977.

_____. *New Mind, New Body.* New York: Harper and Row, 1974.
Authoritative material on biofeedback, including clinical applications, by an expert in the field. Mostly straightforward, with a few references to attainment of altered states of consciousness.

Cade, C. Maxwell, and Coxhead, Nona. *The Awakened Mind: Biofeedback and the Development of Higher States of Awareness.* New York: Delacorte Press, 1979. A vivid example of the promotion of biofeedback to induce altered states of consciousness and psychic experience.

Carter, Mildred. *Hand Reflexology: Key to Perfect Health.* West Nyack, N. Y.: Parker Publishing Co., 1975.

_____. *Helping Yourself with Foot Reflexology.* West Nyack, N. Y.: Parker Publishing Co., 1969.
Primary texts on how to cure everything by pressing on the appropriate parts of the hands or feet. Amazingly comprehensive, considering how far-fetched this therapy is. There are even techniques for developing ESP and exorcising unwanted spirits.

Clark, Linda. *Help Yourself to Health.* New York: Pyramid Books, 1972. What looks like a benign self-help book is loaded with hard-core spiritism and much more. How to develop psychic abilities, find a spirit guide and heal with universal energy. The uninitiated reader who casually brings this book home from the health-food store is in for a surprise.

Green, Elmer and Alyce. *Beyond Biofeedback.* New York: Delacorte Press, 1977. A pioneer team in biofeedback research broadens the horizon for this instrument. Deep forays into meditation, psychic powers and altered states.

Ichazo, Oscar. *Arica Psycho-calisthenics.* New York: Simon and Schuster, 1976. How to exercise your way to spiritual enlightenment. Heavy mystical content to the bodily movements. The favorite "exercise break" of many holistic health conferences.

Jensen, Bernard. *Nature Has a Remedy*. Published by the author, 1978. From the popularizer of iridology, a comprehensive collection of cures from foods, herbs and good thoughts. The material is typical of the health-food subculture, though not necessarily reliable.

——————————. *The Science and Practice of Iridology*. Provo, Utah: Bi World Publishers, 1952. Dr. Jensen's textbook of the science which has yet to be validated in the mainline scientific community.

Karlins, Marvin, and Andrews, Lewis. *Biofeedback: Turning on the Power of Your Mind*. New York: Warner Books, 1973. An example of a popularized study of a technique—with strong emphasis on the sensational. Lots of promises on the back cover, including gaining total control of one's health, behavior and destiny.

Lane, Alice. *The Opening of an Eye*. New York: Zebra Books, 1975. "The amazing new book that reveals how the zodiac rules your cell salts." A peculiar blend of astrology and biochemistry.

Life Energies

Coddington, Mary. *In Search of the Healing Energy*. New York: Destiny Books, 1978. A concise study of universal energy as it has been understood through the ages. One of a series of Warner/Destiny paperbacks on various mystical and occultic themes. The book ends with a strong New-Age scenario of a future in which the Baha'i faith has been universally accepted and individuals "see themselves as developing spirits within a collective, universal evolution of consciousness."

Gordon, Richard. *Your Healing Hands: The Polarity Experience*. Santa Cruz, Calif.: Unity Press, 1978. An illustrated textbook of polarity therapy, one of the lesser-known but overtly mystical ways of manipulating the life-force.

Krieger, Dolores. *The Therapeutic Touch*. Englewood Cliffs, N. J.: Prentice-Hall, 1979. A textbook on the use of therapeutic touch to direct healing energies. Has a strong New Consciousness theme.

Motoyama, Hiroshi. *Science and the Evolution of Consciousness: Chakras, Ki, and Psi*. Brookline, Mass.: Autumn Press, 1978. A serious effort to link scientific research and Eastern mysticism. Dr. Motoyama is determined to develop a unifying theory relating chakras, prana, Ch'i, meridians, psychic phenomena and altered states of consciousness. This is a survey volume, useful if one wishes to experience the thinking of a genuine, New-Age mystical scientist (or scientific mystic).

Schwarz, Jack. *Human Energy Systems*. New York: E. P. Dutton, 1980. The cover says, "A way of good health, using our auric fields—including special eye exercises, a tarot system, and guide to medicinal herbs." Full-blown occult science from a committed psychic healer.

_____. *Voluntary Controls: Exercises for Creative Meditation and for Activating the Potential of the Chakras.* New York: E. P. Dutton, 1978. A companion volume to *Human Energy Systems.*

White, John, and Krippner, Stanley, eds. *Future Science: Life Energies and the Physics of Paranormal Phenomena.* New York: Anchor Books, 1977. This extensive anthology contains dozens of key articles on universal energy. A strong effort to link quantum physics and the occult.

Chinese Medicine

Austin, Mary. *The Textbook of Acupuncture Therapy.* New York: ASI Publishers, 1972. A textbook of classical acupuncture, designed to lead the beginner to a sophisticated knowledge of Ch'i manipulation. Very detailed, it contains exercises and problems for the aspiring therapist. A surprising demonstration of how technical a mystical system can become.

Capra, Fritjof. *The Tao of Physics.* Boulder, Colo.: Shambhala Publications, 1976. The classic attempt to forge a bond between Eastern mysticism and modern physics. A key work in the literature of the New Consciousness.

Diamond, John. *Behavioral Kinesiology: How to Activate Your Thymus and Increase Your Life Energy.* New York: Harper and Row, 1979. How everything from synthetic underwear to CB radios affects the flow of life energy. Now entitled *Your Body Doesn't Lie.*

Krippner, Stanley, and Rubin, Daniel, eds. *The Kirlian Aura: Photographing the Galaxies of Life.* Garden City, N. Y.: Anchor Books, 1974.

_____. *The Energies of Consciousness: Explorations in Acupuncture, Auras and Kirlian Photography.* New York: Gordon and Breach Science Publishers, 1975.

Presentations from the First and Second Western Hemisphere Conferences on Kirlian Photography, Acupuncture and the Human Aura. Each contains highly technical data and highly mystical perspectives.

McGarey, William A. *Acupuncture and Body Energies.* Phoenix, Ariz.: Gabriel Press, 1974. Perspectives on acupuncture and the flow of life energy from a physician committed to the application of Edgar Cayce's readings.

Mann, Felix. *Acupuncture: The Ancient Chinese Art of Healing and How It Works Scientifically.* New York: Random House, 1963. An interesting and detailed handbook on acupuncture theory and practice by a man who does not subscribe to the mysticism of the ancients.

Muramotot, Naboru. *Healing Ourselves.* New York: Avon Books, 1973. A comprehensive handbook on oriental medicine and mysticism. Everything explained in terms of yin and yang. Example: a long nose is a sign of strong yin in the body; a short nose, yang. Lots of herbal and food therapies based on these principles.

Teeguarden, Iona. *Acupressure Way of Health: Jin Shin Do.* Tokyo: Japan Publications, 1978. Heavy psychic technology using acupressure techniques.

Thie, John. *Touch for Health.* Marina del Rey, Calif.: DeVorss and Publishers, 1973. The "new approach to restoring our natural energies" which can bring practical Taoism into anyone's living room. A popular mix of classical Chinese medicine and chiropractic.

Veith, Ilza, trans. *The Yellow Emperor's Classic of Internal Medicine.* Berkeley, Calif.: Univ. of California Press, 1949. The sourcebook for classical Chinese medicine. Ilza Veith's introduction is excellent.

Psychic Healing and Healers

Boyd, Doug. *Rolling Thunder.* New York: Dell Publishing Co., 1974. A firsthand study of a modern American shaman (medicine man), complete with healings, rainmaking, psychic transportation of objects through the air and more.

Cocciardi, Carol; Cocciardi, Mary; Erickson, Karen; and Erickson, Linda, eds. *The Psychic Yellow Pages.* Saratoga, Calif.: Out of the Sky, 1977. An annotated guide to the psychics, astrologers, tarot readers and New-Age healers in northern California.

Fuller, John. *Arigo: Surgeon of the Rusty Knife.* New York: Thomas Crowell Co., 1974. John Fuller's excellent and compelling biography of Arigo.

Joy, W. Brugh. *Joy's Way.* Los Angeles: J. P. Tarcher, 1979. Very intense New-Age metaphysics from a very intense metaphysician.

Krippner, Stanley, and Villoldo, Alberto. *The Realms of Healing.* Millbrae, Calif.: Celestial Arts, 1976. Studies and descriptions of psychic healers by two who believe in them. Includes a section which attempts to explain how psychic healing may work.

LeShan, Lawrence. *The Medium, the Mystic, and the Physicist.* New York: Random House, Ballantine Books, 1975. LeShan's important account of his experiments in training psychic healers.

Meek, George, ed. *Healers and the Healing Process.* Wheaton, Ill.: Theosophical Publishing House, 1977. An extensive anthology dealing with psychic healers of all types, with a fairly heavy New-Age slant.

Miller, Roberta DeLong. *Psychic Massage.* New York: Harper and Row, Harper Colophon Books, 1975. Hard-core psychic orientation. Manipulation of energy flows, auras, past-life material and more, from a mainstream publisher.

Mishlove, Jeffrey. *The Roots of Consciousness*. New York: Random House, The Bookworks, 1975. A tour of the paranormal realm by a knowledge-able and literate guide. This is a comprehensive survey with a definite slant: the reader is given an overt invitation to explore the psychic realm. Lots of interesting pictures and drawings.

Montgomery, Ruth. *Born to Heal*. New York: Popular Library, 1973. From a prolific explorer of the psychic realm, a biography of the anonymous Mr. A, whose psychic healing abilities originated from the "Power of Powers." The author's agreement not to name this gentleman and the frequent references to the "Universal Ring of Wisdom" create an air of unreality despite the many details.

Moss, Thelma. *The Probability of the Impossible*. New York: New Ameri-can Library, 1975. Thelma Moss's investigation into parapsychology and Kirlian photography. Covers the gamut from acupuncture to spirit possession and calls for scientific explorations of the occult realm.

Ostrander, Sheila, and Schroeder, Lynn. *Psychic Discoveries behind the Iron Curtain*. Englewood Cliffs, N. J.: Prentice-Hall, 1970. An entertain-ing if credulous look at Soviet forays into the paranormal. This book contains something for everyone: astrology, ESP, pyramid power and vital energies. Probably outdated now.

The Paul Solomon Tapes. Virginia Beach, Va.: Fellowship of the Inner Light, 1974. Verbatim transcriptions of unconscious readings by a con-temporary sleeping prophet. Rambling discourses on everything from sex to Atlantis, loaded with New-Age themes and thinking. Only the most dedicated would seem able to wade through this muddied dis-course.

Playfair, Guy Lyon. *The Unknown Power*. New York: Pocket Books, 1975. A British author's account of all sorts of psychic occurrences in Brazil, observed over a two-year period. Concludes that we should make a de-termined effort to contact discarnate entities.

Regush, Nicholas M., ed. *Frontiers of Healing: New Dimensions in Para-psychology*. New York: Avon Books, 1977. An anthology of articles by familiar New-Age reporters on familiar New-Age topics. The book be-gins with a commercial for the Academy of Parapsychology and Medi-cine.

_____. *The Human Aura*. New York: Berkeley Corporation, 1974. An anthology of reports on the aura, the luminous glow which psychics claim to see around all of us. Documents attempt to tie this age-old concept to Kirlian photography and modern physics. The cover shows a man and woman, surrounded by a Kirlianlike flare, on the verge of a sensuous kiss, and promises that you can "unlock your own hidden powers to improve your health, emotional well-being, personal relationships, career, and every aspect of your life."

Reilly, Harold J., and Brod, Ruth Hagy. *The Edgar Cayce Handbook for Health through Drugless Therapy.* New York: Macmillan Publishing, 1975. All sorts of advice from the physical therapist who was named hundreds of times in the Cayce readings

Sherman, Harold. *"Wonder" Healers of the Philippines* Santa Monica, Calif.: DeVorss and Co., 1967. Despite the title suggesting uncritical belief in the Filipino psychic surgeons, the author presents as much evidence of fraud as of genuine healing. One of the earliest (1967) accounts of Tony Agpaoa.

Stearn, Jess. *Edgar Cayce, The Sleeping Prophet.* New York: Doubleday, 1967. A popularized biography of Edgar Cayce written by a popularizer of psychic phenomena.

Stelter, Alfred. *Psi-Healing.* New York: Bantam Books, 1976. "Fantastic Medical Cures being performed daily by psychic healers around the world." A German author's rhapsodic account of psychic healers.

Sugrue, Thomas. *There Is a River.* New York: Holt, Rinehart and Winston, 1942.

——————————. *Stranger in the Earth.* New York: Holt, Rinehart and Winston, 1948.
The most literate accounts of Edgar Cayce's life and thinking.

Wallace, Amy, and Henkin, Bill. *The Psychic Healing Book: How to Develop Your Psychic Potential Safely, Simply, Effectively.* New York: Delacorte Press, 1978. Designed to lead the masses into hard-core psychic technology. Includes instructions on contacting your spirit guide, reading past lives, and more.

Worrall, Ambrose A., and Worrall, Olga N. *The Gift of Healing.* New York: Harper and Row, 1965.

——————————. *Explore Your Psychic World.* New York: Harper and Row, 1970.
Stories and theories of psychic healing from the Worralls.

Books on Health and Healing without a New Age World View

Allen, David E.; Bird, Lewis P.; and Herrmann, Robert, eds. *Whole-Person Medicine: An International Symposium.* Downers Grove, Ill.: InterVarsity Press, 1980. Papers describing medicine for whole persons, given at the conference sponsored by the Christian Medical Society and Oral Roberts University. Written from a Christian perspective.

Barnard, Christiaan, ed. *The Body Machine.* New York: Crown Publishers, 1981. A stimulating, pictorial, coffee-table book which touches on numerous subjects in health and disease.

Cooper, Kenneth. *The Aerobics Program for Total Well Being,* New York:

M. Evans and Company, 1982. The most comprehensive of Dr. Cooper's books concerning the value of aerobic exercise. More recently, Dr. Cooper has written *Running Without Fear* (New York: M. Evans and Company, 1985) in response to public concern over running arising from the untimely death of James Fixx. This book stresses the appropriate precautions which should be taken prior to and during a running program.

Cousins, Norman. *Anatomy of an Illness.* New York: W. W. Norton and Company, 1979. A literate and thoughtful account of a serious illness with important implications. Cousins's reflections found their way into the *New England Journal of Medicine.* He also appears on the holistic health speaking circuit, but has been known to criticize from the podium the overbearing mysticism of such gatherings.

Doyle, Rodger P., and Redding, James L. *The Complete Food Handbook.* New York: Grove Press, 1976. A no-nonsense look at foods and nutrition (which makes this book an oasis in the desert).

Graham, M. F. *Inner Energy.* New York: Sterling Publishing Co., 1979. Dr. Graham's superb study of the problem of chronic fatigue. We have prescribed this book enough times to make it a national best seller.

Hansel, Tim. *When I Relax I Feel Guilty.* Elgin, Ill.: David C. Cook, 1979. A multitude of insights in living life to the fullest. Highly recommended.

Larson, Bruce. *There's a Lot More to Health Than Not Being Sick.* Waco, Tex.: Word Publishers, 1981. Selected topics on lifestyle and health, including relationships, goals and general enthusiasm for life. Many worthwhile ideas from a biblical perspective.

MacNutt, Francis. *Healing.* Notre Dame, Ind.: Ave Maria Press, 1974.
————————— *The Power to Heal.* Notre Dame, Ind.: Ave Maria Press, 1977. Food for thought on Christian healing from an articulate Catholic priest.

McMillen, S. I. *None of These Diseases.* Old Tappan, N. J.: Fleming Revell, 1963. A classic of sorts on the relationship between behavior and disease, with insights from the Scriptures.

Minirth, Frank B., and Meier, Paul D. *Happiness Is a Choice.* Grand Rapids, Mich.: Baker Book House, 1978. A comprehensive and informative (yet very readable) study of depression, written from a scientific and biblical viewpoint.

Selye, Hans. *Stress without Distress.* New York: Lippincott Co., 1974.
————————— *The Stress of Life.* New York: McGraw-Hill, 1956. Two classic works on stress by perhaps the most respected authority on the subject. The newer work makes a strong point: stress is not something to be avoided, but to be used as a positive force in life.

Tubesing, Donald A. *Wholistic Health: A Whole-Person Approach to Primary Health Care.* New York: Human Sciences Press, 1979. An excellent and comprehensive study of whole-person medicine without a shred of mysticism. Tubesing served as executive vice-president for the Wholistic Health Centers in Illinois founded by Granger Westberg.

Vickery, Donald M., and Fries, James F. *Take Care of Yourself: A Consumer's Guide to Medical Care.* Reading, Mass.: Addison-Wesley, 1976. One of the best resources around for intelligent home care of medical problems.

Wholesome Diet. Chicago, Ill.: Time-Life Books, 1981. One of the excellent series in the Time-Life Library of Health. Readable text and terrific graphics.

Wholistic Health Centers, 137 S. Garfield Ave., Hinsdale, IL 60521. Anyone seriously interested in whole-person care should write for a list of the excellent monographs and manuals which summarize over a decade of pioneering work by this organization.

Critiques

Consumers Union. *Health Quackery.* New York: Holt, Rinehart and Winston, 1980.

——————————— *The Medicine Show.* Rev. ed. Mount Vernon, N. Y.: Random House, Pantheon Books, 1980.

Straightforward accounts of remedies, useful and otherwise, from the editors of *Consumer Reports.* Good research and fairness all around, in our opinion.

Deutsch, Ronald M. *The New Nuts among the Berries: How Nutrition Nonsense Captured America.* Palo Alto, Calif.: Bull Publishing Company, 1977. This well-researched book is a wickedly funny account of nutritional misinformation over the past century. Be warned: there are no sacred cows in this volume.

Flammonde, Paris. *The Mystic Healers.* New York: Stein and Day, 1974. An entertaining, literate and very hard-nosed look at a gamut of healers. Mr. Flammonde shreds healing claims without regard to race, creed or national origin. His chapter on Christian Science is worth the price of the book. Highly recommended.

Nolen, William A. *Healing: A Doctor in Search of a Miracle.* New York: Random House, 1974. An interesting and important personal assessment of psychic healing. Nolen, a general surgeon, provides an excellent discussion of alternative explanations for miraculous cures.

North, Gary. *None Dare Call It Witchcraft.* Westport, Conn.: Arlington House Publishers, 1976. This is an intelligent analysis of current trends in the psychic and occult realms, written from a biblical slant. Chapters on Edgar Cayce and Arigo are excellent, but the scope of this book is much broader. Retitled *Unholy Spirits* (Dominion Press, 1986)

Sire, James W. *The Universe Next Door.* Downers Grove, Ill.: InterVarsity Press, 1976. Requried reading for an understanding of popular world views. Contains what is perhaps the most lucid discussion in print of the New Consciousness.

The Skeptical Inquirer. The journal of the Committee for the Scientific Investigation of Claims of the Paranormal. Interesting material from a naturalistic/humanistic perspective. Available by writing P.O. Box 29, Kensington Station, Buffalo, NY 14215.

The Spiritual Counterfeits Project. An important resource for thoughtful analysis of current trends in the New Consciousness, paranormal research, cults and numerous other topics. SCP's April 1978 *Journal* was the first critique of the holistic health movement from a biblical perspective. All kinds of valuable articles and essays are available. For current listings and ongoing mailings, write to P.O. Box 4308, Berkeley, CA 94704.

Stalker, Douglas and Glymour, Clarks, eds. *Examining Holistic Medicine.* Buffalo, New York: Prometheus Books, 1985. This is an outstanding anthology of articles critical of the holistic movement from a strictly secular viewpoint. The materials range from general critiques of holistic philosphy and methodology to evaluations of specific practices, including the following: homeopathy, iridology, acupuncture, chiropractic, Therapeutic Touch, visualization treatment for cancer, herbal medicine and biofeedback. Highly recommended for the serious student of New Age medicine.

Weldon, John, and Wilson, Clifford. *Psychic Forces and Occult Shock* Chattanooga, TN: Global Publisher, 1987. A detailed critique of the entire realm of the New Consciousness and the occult from a Christian point of view. Covers the gamut, including Hinduism and yoga, astrology, UFOs, TM, reincarnation, est and a critical look at parapsychology.

Weldon, John, and Levitt, Zola. *Is There Life after Death?* Irvine, Calif.: Harvest House Publishers, 1977. A study of the life-after-life movement led by Drs. Raymond Moody and Elisabeth Kübler-Ross. Written from a biblical viewpoint.

———————. *Psychic Healing.* Chicago, Ill.: Moody Press, 1982. A detailed account of psychic healing written from a Christian perspective.

Subject Index

Index of Names

Helps and Indices of Major Critiques and Analyses
(Page numbers are noted after each reference)

Major Therapies

1. Acupuncture, Acupressure — 58-78, 172-174
2. Applied Kinesiology (Touch for Health, Behavioral Kinesiology, "muscle testing" — 80-89
3. Biofeedback —135-137
4. Chiropractic — 20-22, 37, 44, 48, 52, 80-81, 94, 142, 148-149, 176-177
5. Homeopathy — 137-141
6. Iridology — 141-146
7. Psychic diagnosis, healing, surgery — 97-121
8. Therapeutic Touch — 44-48

Ten Precepts of New Age Medicine

1. The whole is greater than the sum of its parts — 14-16
2. Health is more than the absence of disease — 16-17
3. Individuals are ultimately responsible for their own health or disease — 17-19
4. Natural forms of healing are preferable to drugs and surgery — 19-20
5. Some methods of promoting health and preventing disease are more "holistic" than others — 20-26
6. Health implies evolution — 26-28
7. We need an alternative model of health based on energy rather than matter — 28-30
8. Death is the final stage of growth — 30
9. Ancient civilizations possess a storehouse of knowledge for healty living — 30-31
10. New Age medicine should be integrated into the mainstream through influencing public policy — 31-32

Five Precepts Concerning "Universal Energy" in New Age Medicine

1. "Universal energy" is the basic fabric of everything in the universe 35-37

2. Disease results from a blockage or imbalance in the flow of energy in the body — 37
3. "Universal energy" can be activated or channeled by a healer, and may be for constructive or destructive action — 37-38
4. Alterations in "univesal energy" are the basis for all events which have previously been called supernatural or miraculous — 38-39
5. "Universal energy" is what religions have called God — 39-40

Three Versions of "Universal Energy"

1. Prana (Hinduism) — 40-42, 44-47
2. Mana (shamanism) — 42-44
3. Ch'i (Taoism) — 56-60

Four Basic Principles of New Age Metaphysics
(See pp. 48-59)

1. All is One.
2. We are divine beings.
3. The purpose of life is to become aware of our divine nature.
4. Enlightenment leads to the exercise of "psychospiritual" power.

Nine Priciples for Discernment
(See pp. 148-152)

1. Beware of therapies which claim to manipulate "invisible energy."
2. Beware of those who seem to utilize psychic knowledge or power.
3. Beware of a practitioner who has a therapy with which no one else is familiar.
4. Beware of someone who claims that his or her particular therapy will cure anything.
5. Beware of someone whose explanations don't make sense.
6. Beware of therapies whose primary proof consists of the testimonies of satisfied customers.
7. Beware of therapies which rely heavily on altered states of consciousness.

8. Sincerity is no guarantee of legitimacy.
    Corollary A: A therapist's expression of evangelical commitment is no guarantee of legitimacy.
    Corollary B: The endorsement of a therapy by an evangelical pastor, speaker, author or celebrity is no guarantee of legitimacy.
9. Let the seller beware: i.e., those who offer practices which are unsound or dangerous are ultimately accountable to their patients.

Four Metaphysical Elements of Ancient Chinese Medicine

1. The Tao   54
2. Yin and Yang   54-56
3. Ch'i   56-60
4. The Five Elements   60-62

Critiques of Five Psychic Healers

1. Olga Worrall   101-103
2. W. Brugh Joy   103-105
3. Lawrence LeShan   105-108
4. Arigo   108-112
5. Edgar Cayce   112-121

Examples of Potential Physical Hazards of New Age Medicine

1. In rejecting more appropriate treatment   19-20
2. In behavioral kinesiology   87
3. In homeopathy   141
4. In iridology   145
5. In chiropractic   177

Examples of Potential Spiritual Hazards in New Age Medicine

1. In psychic healing   129-132, 146, 148
2. In theological discernment—preface, 24-26, 39-40, 93-95, 114-116, 126
3. In chiropractic: adding New Age mysticism to legitimate therapy.

204

List of Charts

OTHER BOOKS FROM GLOBAL PUBLISHERS

ISBN NUMBER	DESCRIPTION	UNIT PRICE
0-937931-04-7	*A VOICE FROM HEAVEN* by Ralph W. Neighbour, Sr.	5.95p
0-937931-10-1	*AIDS: YOU THINK YOU'RE SAFE* by Moody Adams	7.95p
0-937931-42-X	*CULTS AT THE CLOSE OF THE 80'S* M. Thomas Starkes	6.95p
0-937931-01-2	*DUAL MINISTRY* by M. Thomas Starkes	3.95p
0-937931-15-2	*EYEWITNESSES OF HIS MAJESTY* Ralph W. Neighbour, Sr.	6.95p
0-937931-00-4	*FAITH BROKERS* by Wally Metts	5.95p
0-937931-08-X	*FREEMASONRY* by Jack Harris	6.95p
0-937931-11-X	*HOLDING THE FORT OR 50 EVENINGS WITH MOODY* by Moody	7.95p
0-937931-07-1	*FUTURE CHURCH* by Ralph W. Neighbour, Jr.	6.95p
0-937931-12-8	*JOHN JASPER* by William E. Hatcher	3.95p
0-937931-27-6	*NEW AGE MEDICINE* by Paul C. Reisser, M.D.,Teri K. Reisser, John Weldon	6.95p
0-937931-09-8	*PSYCHIC FORCES AND OCCULT SHOCK* by John Weldon and C. Wilson	10.95p
0-937931-13-6	*THE REAL BILLY SUNDAY* by E.P. Brown	6.95p
0-937931-03-9	*THE SHINING LIGHT* by Ralph W. Neighbour, Sr.	5.95p
0-937931-05-5	*THE SEARCHING HEART* by Ralph W. Neighbour, Sr.	5.95p
0-937931-06-3	*THINE ENEMY* by Ralph W. Neighbour, Sr.	5.95p

(PRICES SUBJECT TO CHANGE)